fish dreams

A Mother's Journey

From Curing Her Son's Autism

to Loving Him as He Is

IRMA VELASQUEZ

Fish Dreams
A Mother's Journey From Curing Her Son's Autism to Loving Him as He Is
Irma Velasquez
Deep Living Lab, Inc.

Published by Deep Living Lab, Inc., San Mateo, CA

Editor: Jeannette Encinias, Book Coach, www.jeannetteencinias.com
Cover and Interior design: Davis Creative, CreativePublishingPartners.com

Publisher's Cataloging-In-Publication Data
(Provided by Cassidy Cataloguing Services, Inc.)

Names: Velasquez, Irma, author.
Title: Fish dreams : a mother's journey from curing her son's autism to loving him as he is / Irma Velasquez.
Description: San Mateo, CA : Deep Living Lab, Inc., [2022] | Includes bibliographical references.
Identifiers: ISBN: 979-8-9860193-0-7 (paperback) | 979-8-9860193-1-4 (ebook) | LCCN: 2022907290
Subjects: LCSH: Parents of autistic children--Biography. | Autistic children--Family relationships. | Autism--Treatment. | Mothers and sons. | Parenting. | LCGFT: Autobiographies. | BISAC: BIOGRAPHY & AUTOBIOGRAPHY / People with Disabilities. | FAMILY & RELATIONSHIPS / Autism Spectrum Disorders. | PHILOSOPHY / Mind & Body.
Classification: LCC: RJ506.A9 V45 2022 | DDC: 618.92858820092--dc23

Dedication

For Aaron, whose wisdom guides me.

For Sherman, who holds the light.

For my parents Jorge and Irma
who nestled me in their hearts.

Acknowledgements

This memoir has been gestating within me for many years. I want to acknowledge many who have nurtured the seedling and encouraged me along the way.

Many years ago, my dear friend, Victoria Jackson, planted the seed for this book and ushered the first few pages into the world. I wish you could be here to share it with me.

I express my gratitude to those who have shared countless hours and contributed their kind and honest feedback. Special thanks to Susan Kinsella and Carolyn Curtis, my steady writing companions. And to Susan for her work on organizing and researching the content of the Book Notes.

I thank my editor, Jeannette Encinias, who kept me on track and inspired me with her poetry and love. And those who edited the final manuscript; Theresa Rogers, Victress Hitchcock, Susan Rogers, who offered their thoughtful insights.

I've come to share a deep respect for those who have stepped courageously into the grounds of education and whose selfless dedication brings hope to our world. To Patty McCague, who lovingly volunteered to be Aaron's first teacher, Liz Jordan, who gave time so freely during his inclusive years in the Kindergarten classroom, and Danielle Thorp Sutton, who shared her love with Aaron in the playroom.

Special thanks to those who braved through the beginning of a Wings Learning Center: Manuela Seitz Hipkins, Jaejin Lee, Kathy Small, Amy Travers, Kara Grant, Rene Trimarco, Mitra Ahani, Andrew Shahan, Dr. Adriana Schuler, Dr. Pamela Wolfberg and many, many more that shared their vision and spent hours in the classroom. Each one brought their gifts and passion for forming a school that values the student as the source of wisdom. To Safa Rashtchy, who Chaired the Board of Directors through years of growth and expansion, Karen Kaplan steered the school towards a sustainable future. To the many parents who taught me valuable lessons in resilience and trust and provided countless resources.

I'm grateful for my friends and colleagues who opened my heart and allowed me to step firmly on the ground of reality: Desiree Goyette for her guidance during the early years of motherhood, Dr. Roxanne Howe-Murphy, my teacher, mentor, and soul sister that has guided me through my inner evolutionary journey. To my Deep Living Circle soul mates; Jean Blomo, Rosie Picchi, Jeannene Minnix Kingston, Bernadette McAllister, Alexandra Subramanian, Kristi Koberna, Christine Portman, Elizabeth Switzer and Samuel Schindler. To my PDS sisters who have been my companions through my inner journey; Dr. Karen Van Zino, Lara Heller, Susan Hansch, Devon Carter, and Dr. Ipek Serifsoy. And to my Deep Living Lab partners, Marcia Hyatt, Liz Vanderwerff, and Barbara Mathison. To Dr. Belinda Gore for opening the door to the wisdom available through the world of alternate realities.

I offer heartfelt gratitude to the health care professionals who work tirelessly to find treatment options for those with autism. A special thanks to Dr. David Traver, Dr. Vicky Cruz, Jana Axelrad, and Dr. Hellen Alderson. And to the many who I have not mentioned in these pages.

There are many to whom I owe immense gratitude; without them, I would not have finished this book. Especial thanks to those who have cared for Aaron through the years and guided him: Pat Conlin, who stepped in during Aaron's formative years and connected with him through her loving heart, Laxmi Ghale, who invited Aaron to gain more and more confidence in himself; Robert Lopez, who led Aaron into his early years of adulthood,

Susana Alcaraz, whose loving care is a source of comfort. And to those who are not named here but remain in our hearts.

And to my parents, through whom I experience the holding environment of a family structure. And to my extended family for their continued love and support.

Lastly, I want to thank my life partner, Dr. Sherman Chan, whose patience, love, wisdom, brilliance, and generous spirit sweeten each moment of the life we share.

Table of Contents

Preface

Intention

All my life I've lived close to the Pacific Ocean, within miles or just over a low mountain ridge. As I've moved North—from El Salvador where I was born, to the San Francisco Bay Area where I've lived all my adult life—the ocean has been consistently within twenty or so miles from the places I've called home.

As a child, I found safety in the sandy beaches, salty waters, and ocean breezes, surrounded by family and friends, always ending our weekend outings with a walk down the pier where fishermen untangled flapping tails from nets brimming with the day's catch. A bountiful ocean has been a constant reminder of the generosities of life.

I started this book after my world began to crumble, and both safety and generosity unfolded into fear. Unanswered questions left me paralyzed: Why is my son not developing like other children? Why is he broken? How do I repair the damage? These unanswered questions left me fearful, insecure, and distrusting of the world around me, and not even the ocean could bring me peace.

My search for a knowing that did not exist, the cure or treatment of autism, led me towards a deeper level of knowing that required me to look inside myself and ask the questions I share with you in these pages.

When we received the diagnosis in 1997, my husband and I were told autism was a rare and incurable disease, affecting three in every ten thousand children. As I write this preface, the statistics are very different. Now you will find many personal accounts from mothers and autistic individuals who articulate their plight with courage and specificity. Research in the far-reaching fields of genetic mapping, brain plasticity, gastrointestinal diseases, and autoimmune responses, to name a few, have advanced our knowledge of this complex and seemingly once rare disease. The field of education has spurred new methods of teaching children with learning differences, and therapeutic models abound. New pathways of engagement for parents have been opened by abundant information and advancements that were unavailable in the past, when limited knowledge once prevented parents from intervening in the development of their children. Instead, I focus on a different kind of knowing that begins with us as parents.

The image I had of my son began to change, and it evolved into a new sense of myself and the world around me. I learned a new language—one taught in the silence of my own interior and the presence of my son. I began to see him for the incredible human being that he is, and in turn, I began a new relationship with myself and those around me.

This book began as a sort of user's manual, one I wish I had when I first became the mother of an autistic child: a practical book of strategies that would guide other parents when met with the unexpected diagnosis of autism. I've included notes in the back of the book as a guide, based on my experience. However, a more informed message has evolved over the years which can't be found in research papers or double-blind studies. The stories I've chosen to share with you hold a deeper intention. I hope they will be a companion and encourage confidence in yourself. A deeper knowing is within you. A knowing that will illuminate the next step you are meant to take, what direction to move towards, and where to land. This knowing resides within you.

I invite you to trust your own knowing and engage with the anecdotes in these pages in a non-linear journey through unmapped territory. My hope is that you will begin to feel at home in yourself and trust in your inner guidance as a form of support through your parenting journey. Undoubtedly you will face moments of confusion, pain, and unease as you walk through this unfamiliar territory. Note these as signposts for paying attention to your inner messenger, who carries an intelligence only you can recognize.

Poems

I wrote the poems included among the chapters with Aaron's voice in mind. I can only guess how he may express himself if he spoke in words. His voice is unique and does not translate to the written word.

Notes

The notes to each section give you more background behind the topics, people, and terms discussed in the chapters.

Many have inspired me over the years; in the notes, I share their wisdom and hint how you can enrich your journey as you explore theories, studies, methods, and yourself.

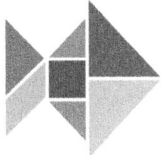

PART 1
Unaccustomed Home

"As soon as they had taken off the mourning clothes for their grandmother, which they wore with inflexible rigor for three years, their bright clothes seemed to have given them a new place in the world."

Gabriel Garcia Marquez,
One Hundred Years of Solitude

Aboard Pan Am Flight 1206

Doors slammed one after the other, and soon a caravan of cars moved in synchronicity towards the Guatemala border. Father was leaving.

"I'll be back soon," he said, and kissed the top of my head. I was nine years old when he left.

Jorge, my brother, dangled out the window, looking back at the line of cars behind ours. It seemed like our entire family was joining the caravan—aunts, abuelas, uncles, cousins—all were going to say goodbye to my father and his fellow travelers on the 3,100-mile trip to California.

It was late March 1963. The day was overcast; dark clouds announced the usual afternoon thunder showers. A quiet stillness settled in our car. Father and Mother sat in the front seat, Jorge and I in the back with Abuela Mirtala, Father's mother, between us, clasping a wet handkerchief in one hand and holding mine with the other. Father's knapsacks were already on top of Romeo's Plymouth station wagon. This was our last trip as a family before we said goodbye.

"When are you coming back?" I asked. I don't know if Father heard my question but I did not ask it again.

Romeo, his wife, and three daughters lived in California where many of Mother's relatives settled in the 1940s. They were heading home to Sebastopol, a farming town in Northern California. Their vacation was over, and they may have been short of cash.

"We have room for one more," Romeo said, somewhat kidding, to my father who jumped at the chance to travel to Los Estados.

"Por supuesto," he said reassuringly, and within a few days gave notice to his boss and packed his bags for an adventure he could not imagine.

"Are you going to stay with Romeo?" I asked as we drove to his destination.

"I'm not sure where I'll be—maybe with your Aunt Consuelo or Uncle Edgar in San Francisco," he said, comfortable with not knowing.

"Will you be back for Mom's birthday?" I asked.

"That's two months away," was all he said. Her birthday was in September, six months away. Father was not known to pay attention to details. I stopped asking. There were too many unanswered questions I couldn't hold.

A dense, green jungle lined the international highway that took us to the border between Guatemala and El Salvador. Jorge knelt on the back seat, counting the cars behind us as I opened the window and stuck my hand out; somehow, maybe I could slow the car down. We drove for hours, but it seemed as if we had just left the city. I leaned my head against the front seat and glanced at my father's slim face and pencil mustache. We sat without saying a word, each of us looking at the road ahead.

The car ahead of us slowed down; we had reached the border. As we came to a stop, two men in green uniforms with machine guns strapped to their backs appeared on each side of the car.

Father turned around and looked at my brother. "Take care of your mother and sister," he said, and ran his fingers through my mother's thick, black hair. Abuela Mirtala dried tears from her eyes and reached for my father's hand, the last time she would touch her son. Cataracts had taken her sight years before.

"Cuidate hijo," she said as she looked straight ahead.

"I'm not leaving until they check the papers," he said, and touched her hand.

We stood outside the car, the four of us, while the soldier walked back to a small office with Father's passport and papers in hand. Abuela waited in the car.

When I saw the soldier walk towards us, I hid my face in my father's bony chest. He smelled like he did when he came home from work—sweaty, with hints of cigarette smoke.

The man in the uniform signaled my father over and pointed to a piece of paper. My father shrugged his shoulders, then walked back to the car. Something was not right.

"¿Que pasa?" Mother asked.

"I don't have the right visa to go into Guatemala," Father said. I noticed a drop of sweat coming down his temple, felt relieved, and could now take a breath.

"Do they want a mordida?" Mother asked. Father was not going to spend his last dollars on a bribe.

"They won't let me go through," Father yelled over to Romeo, who was walking towards us to see what had happened.

Romeo's pale face turned red as he threw his hand in the air and sputtered unintelligible words in English.

On our drive back to San Salvador, I was happy Father was still driving the car and not Uncle Sergio, who had been going to drive us back home. Romeo followed our car but before we entered the city the caravan took a detour to a roadside shack, where we stopped for tamales, pupusas, and quesadillas. I quietly celebrated the mishap.

A few weeks later the scene was repeated, but this time only two cars followed the station wagon to the border. The man in the green uniform seemed to recognize my father and after a few minutes nodded in approval.

We got out of the car and hugged Father goodbye one last time. Then he and his fellow travelers drove away. Jorge and I stood in the middle of the highway, waving to the hands that protruded from both sides of the car like octopus tentacles waving in the wind. I placed my arm around Mother's waist, Jorge held tightly onto her hand. She cried in her quiet manner until the wagon disappeared in the distance.

Two months had passed when we received a telegram from Father: SELL THE HOUSE. SELL THE CAR. BRING THE KIDS.

Mother was a loyal wife who didn't question Father's decisions. She sold everything we owned, including the new bike that had been my birthday present earlier that year. With the proceeds of the sale, she bought plane tickets for the three of us. She left for Los Estados in September of the same year with one thousand dollars in her purse—barely enough to set up a home for the four of us in a new country. Jorge and I waited for our turn.

My brother and I boarded Pan American flight 1206; the flight to San Francisco left at four o'clock on a balmy December afternoon in 1963. Disoriented by the last-minute hugs and tears of the only family I knew, I smelled my abuela's ancient scent one last time as she cradled me tightly against her breast. Her fingertips held onto my sleeve just one more second before she slowly released the tip of my blouse, then reluctantly let go. Then a tall, slim woman wearing a pillbox hat and a dark-blue uniform extended her hand, inviting us to follow her across the tarmac and up the aluminum stairs that led us inside the double-engine plane. Fifty years later, the last-minute calls at airports take me back to that day, when I experienced the first of many unknowns. A pat on the knee and the sound of the seatbelt locking into place invited me into a new reality.

"It's going to be fine, honey. Soon you'll be with your mom and dad," she said, and glanced over with a kind smile.

Of course it was fine; it had always been fine. In my nine-year-old self there was nothing but fine. I held the smile on the lady's face as long as I could and wondered what it was I didn't know.

I put both hands over my ears as the plane began to move down the runway. Engines rumbled, the cabin shook, wheels retracted, and then there was a brief silence. Jorge leaned over close to me as we looked out the tiny window. Down below were faded spots that had once been homes, office buildings, and white churches. They began to transform from rectangles to dots and then to splattered, lightened shades of brown. I imagined my abuelas, tias, and primos, down on the ground crying and comforting each other, telling themselves it was all for a better life in Los Estados.

Did our lives really need to be better? How could they be? Each breath of ocean air deepened the memories; each bite of pine-apple sweetened the faces of those who shared it with me. I already missed the leftover scent of burnt firecrackers on New Year's Day and my grandmother's touch each time I came to see her in her one-bedroom home.

The sun faded on the horizon, and I began to feel uneasy. I adjusted my taffeta skirt, trying to ease the rough edges that prickled against my thighs. I really didn't like the serious-looking outfit Abuela Esther had made for me: a dark-blue blouse and skirt to match. Until then, I hadn't been too particular about what I wore, but this time I felt myself fighting against the grown-up outfit. I wanted to go back to my light, cotton sleeveless dresses with floral prints. But this flight was a special occasion. It was time for a somber wardrobe.

Suddenly a voice came over the speaker. We were now flying over Guatemala. Ahead was the Gulf of Mexico. The sky was turning a deep indigo blue. The ocean was dark and ominous, but in the distance, lights began to twinkle—signs of boats or maybe homes. A terrain I had only seen in textbooks appeared, except that this scene didn't have any borders. All I could see on the horizon was an endless ocean. Suddenly the world seemed immense and limitless.

Darkness covered the terrain for hours until the enchanted city appeared below. Mother had told us about her experience when she flew over the City of Angels. That meant we were almost home, but home had a different meaning now. Free from walls, a roof, or floors, now it was a place that had no place on the map of my consciousness,   but a home, nevertheless, anchored only by my parents. As we walked through the skybridge I saw Mother, tears in her eyes, standing next to Father, whose mustache now covered most of his broad smile. We embraced and welcomed each other home to the cold winter days that were ahead of us.

The next morning, I opened the door to a new world and temperatures I had never experienced before, close to freezing. The streets were empty and gray, with rooftops whitened by frozen dew of the early morning. At the park, people looked at my brother and me as if we were aliens from another planet. San Mateo, a suburb south of San Francisco, was homogeneously white. I now had a new identity; I was different. Years later, the civil rights movement brought home the violent realities of our new homeland. Riots and an assassination in the City of Angels made me wonder if this was the best decision Father could have made.

Those first years in the new country were lonely. The ground beneath me had been moved, and I was trying to establish my foothold on the familiar. A box of photographs kept me company when I felt alone. Blurred black-and-white images taken with my father's 35-mm camera were thrown together in a pink box with more recent color photographs.

In black and white: snap—me, a toddler with my face covered with black volcanic sand. I remembered joyfully rolling around in this fine, soft powder until I could not stand the fine particles in my most intimate crevices. When I ran into the warm ocean, Abuela screamed, "¡Cuidado!"

Next shot, in color: standing next to my new blue bike in front of our home in California—one foot resting on a pedal, the other ready to push myself off to school. That bike cost my mother a day's work of scrubbing toilets and cleaning houses. I never forgot that.

Next shot: Aunt Rose and Christos at church, ready to recite their wedding vows. Behind them, a priest, his hands stretched over their heads. They married a year after we left. I missed being their flower girl.

A black-and-white shot: at the airport. Mother wiping her tears with a white handkerchief, standing at the boarding gate.

Faded color: Jorge and I on the sofa with Cousin Esther, our arms around each other as if we were old friends, sitting in her home overlooking the Pacific Ocean. I was now part of a family I had only experienced in black-and-white photographs. The day we took that picture we had finished watching The Beatles on The Ed Sullivan Show. Screaming girls on the television screen made no sense to me. Nor did my cousin's behavior as she jumped up and down in the living room, shaking her Ringo-style hairdo from side to side. I felt as if I was watching two movies playing, overlapping each other on the screen: one where I was a character in the story and the other where I was sitting in the theater, watching the screen.

Black and white: Father, alone, his tall, thin body bending over, elbow on his knee, his foot on the fender of the Plymouth station wagon, holding his ticket to California. Was he a gambler or an explorer? Did he know he would not return to his homeland for another thirty-five years? Did he portend the political stability that followed in El Salvador in the '80s or fear the spread of communism Castro and Che started in Cuba in 1959? Father never gave me an explanation for his decision. And Mother didn't have the answer.

I was the only one in our family who continued to return to visit the country we left behind, year after year, until all my closest relatives had died and my childhood friends had moved to other countries. Maybe I was waiting or searching for the answers to the question I asked Father the day he left. In my sixties, the questions remain, and I wonder how my life would have been different if my father had not tried to cross the border a second time.

Wooden Angels

My first premonition of motherhood came in the dark, humble home of a prestigious palm reader on the outskirts of San Salvador. My cousin was a believer in these forms of knowledge and far more curious than I was about my future.

"Will I have children?" I asked, not knowing what else to say—a common question in a culture where family is at the center. Something inside me rebelled against the norms—at least for the first thirty-six years.

"I see two, maybe three," the shriveled old man said as he examined my palm with his dark, bony index finger as if analyzing a rare manuscript. Many years later, after several attempts at motherhood, I remembered the palm reader's prediction.

In my teens, I spent my summer vacations in El Salvador, deepening my relationships with the family I had left behind. I longed for my childhood friends—cousins with whom I'd shared my formative years and adults who held me tenderly during my childhood. My life in California was passionless, and since I had no close friendships except for my parents and brother, I fled back to the place where I was born.

Soon after I landed at the Salvadorean airport, I would rush to Abuela Esther's home, anticipating her warm hug. I'd drive up to her house on top of the same dusty street where I grew up and find her leaning out her front window, chatting with the passersby, waiting for me to appear.

"There she is!" she'd say to her companion and abruptly drop the conversation, open the door, and run to meet me. How could I not be close to her? She raised me during the first five years of my life, while my parents both worked to make ends meet. A handsome woman with bronze skin, hazel eyes, and thick, silver hair, she drew me into her arms the moment I saw her. She was not one to sit for long. I followed her around the house as we caught up with the news about family back in *Los Estados*, then to the patio where she tossed morsels of dried tortilla to the turtles that came out from under the rocks when they heard the clicking sound of her leather heels on the tile floor. Her life fascinated me.

I'm still in awe of her ability to birth nine and raise seven children as a single mother. Even though Abuelo Miguel was in the house, he was bed-ridden after a massive stroke and also needed her care. I wanted to know how she did it and would listen to the stories of schemes she contrived to bring food to the table: sewing for the local military billet, inventing new dishes to sell at the local market. As the church artisan, she fashioned garments on wooden angels for the parades through the barrio during Holy Week. A favorite artistic creation was the multicolor sawdust carpet that covered the dusty street in front of her house and blended back into the dust after the procession passed over it.

When Abuela Esther passed at the age of seventy-six, she had buried four of her children. Two had died as toddlers to an unknown childhood disease, a son to a bullet fired by a jealous lover, and her oldest daughter gave in to a sudden heart attack at the age of forty. The first few years of my life with Abuela Esther made me see the cruel realities of life and the beauty and resilience that exists within us, as well as the drive to brave the lessons of time.

I admired her resilience and resourcefulness. For a woman with little education, she had insisted her children have some form of skill or occupation. She lived in the silence of her experiences, not wanting to talk much about her past. I wonder if this was a way of distancing herself from the pain of the losses she experienced in her life. I later asked myself if I wasn't doing the same.

While in my mid-thirties, unmarried and childless, I had given up the idea of having a family in any form. My life path would be different from that of my mother or grandmother. I was determined to avoid Abuela's steps of single-handedly raising even one child without a partner, and marriage seemed more like an obligation than a future. Privileged to be brought up in a two-parent home, I was determined to do the same or not have children at all.

Then I met Sherman.

On our first date, as we walked down to the Rodin sculpture garden on the Stanford campus, a young woman jogger passed us by, pushing a stroller. Sherman suddenly stopped, looked back at her, and gave me a gentle smile. I had just met him—how could he so blatantly stop our conversation to check out a pair of bare legs? I quickly realized he was looking inside the stroller, not at the woman.

"There's a humanoid in there," he said with a smile and looked for my reaction. I relaxed and was charmed by his curiosity and spontaneous response.

Later in our courtship, one morning, still in bed and looking out at the clear sky through the attic window, I became curious.

"Do you want to have children?" I asked, wanting to hear his plans.

"I don't think we should have them until we're married," he responded and proposed at the same time. So, I said yes to motherhood and marriage without saying a word.

In November 1991, we celebrated Sherman's thirty-eighth birthday, our first wedding anniversary, and our future child in Santa Fe, New Mexico; the City of Holy Faith, The Loretto Chapel and adobe homes on cobbled streets reminded me of El Salvador and drew me back years later. Just like my new life as a wife and mother-to-be, the dry desert of the Southwest was new terrain. I left enchanted with the open skies, the reflecting colors of the sunsets against the stone-peaked mountains, and the vulnerable landscape, which bore the harshness of nature. Thin sheets of snow covered the sagebrush on the khaki-colored fields as we took in the dry, open desert.

Gates of Hell

Aftershocks of the Loma Prieta earthquake shook my world on a warm November day in 1989. Security as I knew it was about to change near the rubble of uncertainty that had befallen the San Francisco Bay a few weeks before. A discomfort I had felt all my life when my feet left the ground was now a conscious companion.

Stillness followed the 6.8 jolt on October 17. Muffled news reports came from car radios. A span of the Bay Bridge had fallen, and the thoroughfare to the East Bay was closed. For several months the Bay Area was gridlocked. For me, a new life was about to begin.

I first saw him standing, arms behind his back, at the front entrance to the California Cafe, holding his aviator jacket in one hand as if waiting for a ride. He had an unassuming, casual look. His straight, black hair was slowly disappearing behind short strands of white. His skin was dark except for a few blotches of pink I later learned was eczema. His brown eyes were barely visible amongst his Asian features.

I tried not to be overly apologetic, but was pressed to explain why I was a half-hour late for our first date.

"As I was walking out, the phone rang. Something told me I had to get the call. It was my brother, excited about his newborn daughter," I said, fully aware of doing one-last-thing before leaving the house.

"What's her name?" he asked. He was calm and showed a genuine interest in knowing more about my niece. As we resumed our conversation in the sparse restaurant, our thoughts flowed smoothly from one question to the next.

Over black coffee we began to untangle the web of strangers that had brought us together. Two sisters orchestrated our meeting. Each one knew bits and pieces about each of us. Sherman's college friends chimed in and thought we would make a good match.

"What is he like?" I asked the sister who called me unexpectedly.

"I've actually never met him. But I know his friend," she said, and she began to talk to me about Sherman's college classmate.

"I met Harriet last week for the first time when I picked up my birthday cake," he said as he gulped down a whole egg yolk in one bite.

"Well, happy belated birthday! How many?" I asked.

"Thirty-six, and you?" he said.

"Not far behind you. I'll catch up in January," I replied.

Two strangers introduced me to the man I later married. Hildy and Harriet were proud of their matchmaking skills, having successfully "married off" several friends.

When I think back to that moment, thoughts of my mother return. Oftentimes when she and I were in the throes of a visceral discussion, she knew just what to say to shut me up.

"I know you," she'd say, with a certainty that only a mother could own. Those words infuriated me and made me feel alone and misunderstood. Of course she didn't know me, I thought, as a teenager and as an adult woman. How could she? How could strangers who don't know us be so sure about us? I felt naked with a certainty that they did and I didn't.

As we sat in the Cafe, Sherman continued to talk and I continued to listen, intrigued by the story of how his family immigrated from China to Hong Kong before settling in Portland, Oregon. We exchanged similar experiences of our lives in a new country and shared memories of early school days that were very similar. Kids pushed each other out of the way to get a closer look at the new kid in school. Curious eyes stared at us on the playground. I recalled the laughter that erupted around me when I could not pronounce a word. Sherman nodded; he, too, had been there.

He remembered bussing tables in Uncle Ding's restaurant, earning a dollar an hour, and picking strawberries for three cents a pound, until his fingers turned red. For moments we were living in each other's lives. Our fathers had worked as gardeners and bussed tables, earning minimum wage. Our mothers had had different aspirations. Silvia, Sherman's mom, stayed home to take care of her three sons. He lowered his glance when he began to talk about his mother.

"She died two months ago. She suffered for years from scleroderma," he said in a somber voice. "It's not hereditary," he quickly added.

As we talked, he danced his fingers across the top of the table as if it was the keyboard of a piano, a habit that continues to this day. Music had colored his life as art had mine. He gave me a brief history of his favorite romantic composer, Chopin, and listed his favorite etudes. Embarrassed to admit I knew little about his music, I launched into my love for impressionist artists. We began to talk one language, alternating between music and art.

"I have plans to study art in Florence," I blurted out.

"Aren't you too old for that?" he said. I liked his straight, matter-of-fact response, which left little room to guess what he was thinking. There was a familiarity underneath the worlds where both of our passions rested.

Somehow our experiences in a new country had given us a familiar place from which to start our conversation. Art and music led us towards a deeper exploration of our relationship.

Neither one of us wanted the afternoon to end. I wanted to know more about this mysterious stranger. In some curious and odd way, he seemed very incisive and honest.

"Do you want to see The Gates of Hell?" he asked as he interrupted our walk towards our cars.

"Ummmm, sure," I said, surprised by the sudden question and embarrassed I didn't know what he was talking about.

"The new Rodin sculpture," he said as he acknowledged my hesitation.

In full display amidst the Stanford campus was the Rodin sculpture garden that had been completed just a few years before, in 1985. I felt like an impostor; how did I not know about this? How could I be thinking about Florence and know nothing of Dante, his famous work, The Divine Comedy, or even this treasure of a garden a few minutes from my home?

We walked into a magical garden where massive bronze sculptures rested peacefully outside the Rodin Museum. Two female figures, stooped by the weight on their shoulders, took their place among several standing pieces. I moved towards one and Sherman to the other.

I glanced at Sherman, standing several yards away from me in front of The Fallen Caryatid Carrying Her Stone. The afternoon sun glazed the sculpture with light. He circled it slowly and moved his hand around the voluptuous hips, then over the curved back of the feminine figure. The sensuality of his caress made me move towards him.

"Is this your favorite piece?" I asked.

"Not necessarily. Sculptures like to be felt," he answered, without taking his eyes off the sculpture.

On the other end of the garden was The Gates of Hell, the famous, unfinished work by Rodin. Full figures of Adam and Eve guarded the gate. We walked together towards the masterpiece, which resembled the unfinished façade of a door.

I looked up and pointed at the small sculpture above the entrance.

"The Thinker," I said.

"It's actually called The Poet. It's supposed to be Dante looking down on the bloody mess," Sherman said, and looked at me. For a moment our eyes met as we shared a mutual delight in the depictions of hell before us and the drama within the fold of each figure on the side of the gate: the desperate sinners, Paolo and Francesca—two lovers collapsing into each other's arms, the pain of unfulfilled love earning its place amid other fallen figures. A masterpiece inspired by Dante's journey through hell, purgatory, and finally, heaven.

Sherman explained the story in detail and without any pretense. I moved close to him as we walked around the garden, both of us silently engaged in the drama of each sculpture. It was a private tour through a garden of melted bronze and unknown dreams.

Over the past thirty years, I've replayed that November day over and over in my head. It's been the story I tell those who ask how I met my husband and the father of my child.

I didn't know how our story would unfold or that under the afternoon sun we were recapping our lives together. Somehow, we stepped into a story that was already written, like the autumn leaves on the sycamore trees, which did not have a destination as they fell to the ground that met them below.

Fish Dreams

Mother said that fish dreams were a good omen, especially when you could remember the details. It happened in the middle of the night—I was jerked awake by the vivid details of a dream. Two dim eyes took up most of the panorama inside my head. All I could make out was the gummy film that covered the corneas of a creature that resembled a sizable carp stuffed inside a glass jar. Its half-open mandible opened and closed as if gasping for air as its tail moved rhythmically, touching the sides of the jar. Later that morning, Sherman and I sat in the doctor's office, eagerly awaiting the amnio results.

As we walked out of the doctor's office and into the cold San Francisco morning, I shared the dream with Sherman. We held hands as we ambled to our car, knowing the celebratory lunch we had planned in Chinatown was not going to happen. After seeing the image of my belly on the screen and listening to the doctor's prognosis, it was clear our baby was not going to make it. I felt an unexplainable loss. The unfamiliarity of the situation obscured my emotions. The being inside me was gone before I had the chance to get to know him. My heart was in ruins. Guilt rose as I held the possibility of somehow being responsible for the loss. After all, he was residing in my aging body. I was in my late thirties; my mother had raised two teenagers at my age. Did I have an unconscious hand in its development? This life force had ceased to be a force; it was wilting into formless tissue which held a deep and unfamiliar connection with the rest of me. It took time to recover from the experience.

Months later, I had another fish dream. The body of this fish was long and stiff. Dark, rotting flesh was transforming into a massive black cloud. This charcoal-colored creature lay on its side, on a plank, as if it was the main dish at a fancy meal. It had no eyes; the scene was black, murky, and ominous.

That morning I woke up to blood-stained sheets, a clear sign that what started in my belly only a few weeks before was transforming into another loss. I walked cautiously into the bathroom, bent over with pain, and called Sherman in the only voice I could muster. A visit to the doctor confirmed what I already knew. Yet she encouraged us to continue trying.

"You're not even forty," she said with a reassuring smile.

This second loss didn't deter us from trying for the child that would make us a family. Months later, I walked into the kitchen, eagerly waiting to share a dream with Sherman.

"I had another fish dream," I said.

"Oh, oh!" he said, and placed his cup of coffee on the counter, ready to listen.

"I think this one is going to make it," I said with certainty. Something told me it was a boy; after all, Sherman was one of three brothers. Boys were common in the Chan family—a fact Peter, Sherman's father, proudly recounted.

The fish in this dream was like an acrobat, hanging on a fishline, alive with energy. It dangled from above, a place I couldn't make out in the dream. Its long, majestic tail moved ferociously from left to right, struggling to release itself from captivity. Nine months passed without much drama, as if I was riding a train moving slowly towards an unknown destination. The regular visits to the OB/GYN ended with the exact words from Dr. Cove: "Keep up the good work." I waddled home as we continued to remodel what was once a duplex into a single-family home. The baby's bedroom was bright and open, with a view of a hundred-year-old redwood tree. On the other side was a silk tree with an evergreen canopy covered by delicate red flowers during part of the year. Finally, we refurbished the room next to the nursery into a playroom, ready for his friends to engage in rambunctious play.

Other than a feeling of constant fatigue, I felt no other signs that labor was soon approaching. Thoughts of a possible Cesarean loomed in my subconscious, but Dr. Cove assured me it was unlikely; it was going to be a natural birth. The due date came and went without any signs of contractions or pain. So, each night before going to bed, I caressed my belly as Sherman played Chopin in the living room, wondering if my son would be a dancer, a musician, or maybe an artist of some kind. When he was ten days overdue, we had no choice but to induce.

"He sure doesn't want to come out into the world," one nurse said.

"He has a strong heart," another nurse assured me.

Things began to happen when the nurse introduced the epidural. We started the work of getting the little being out into the world, with encouragement from the nurses and physical help from petite Dr. Cove. She stood on a stool to reach the top of my belly and placed her whole weight against my stomach as the nurses shouted in unison:

"Push!"

Hours later, there he was. One eye was open, and the other one closed. His milky skin was warm and pale; black, abundant hair covered his scalp. His eyes were round, unlike his father; brown, unlike mine. The only sign of his Asian genes was the straight, black hair that almost covered his one wide-open eye. Not a sound came from his half-open lips that mirror Sherman's full lips shaped like small pieces of tangerine. The warmth of his seven-pound body felt at home on top of my belly. Perhaps tired from the twelve-hour journey, we rested together.

The Angst Box

As soon as I met my son, Aaron, we were separated. We'd shared an intimate space for nine months. His heart was mine, and mine his. My skin melted into his just for a few seconds, then the nurse took him away. When she brought him back, looking like a tightly-wrapped cocoon with a makeshift hat, I was in love. His birth was an event of the wills: his body against mine. A twelve-hour journey for him; for me, one of a lifetime. I was thirty-nine when Aaron was born. Until then, I had never really thought about my body or the capacity within me.

"Choose a date. We can't wait much longer," Dr. Cove had said during my last checkup visit. Aaron was ten days overdue, and I had felt no signs of contractions.

"Six, three, nine—all good numbers," Sherman had said while looking at the calendar on her desk.

"Next week it is," Dr. Cove had said.

The long-awaited contractions never came and my water didn't break, so I gave in to modern medicine to help me get my baby out into the world. The night before his birth date, we checked into the hospital room, and as we shared Chinese food from our favorite restaurant on Geary Street, a meal of salt-baked chicken, we talked about how our lives were about to change.

Let me say this about this life-changing experience: I'm recollecting these experiences twenty-some years after they happened, yet the memories I'm about to share are as vivid as if they happened yesterday and carry emotional energy that has an important message.

It was 6:00 a.m. when I woke up to clinks and wheels screeching into the room. Nurses began to transform the hospital suite into a delivery room. IV tubing dangled from metal carriers; stirrups and handles appeared somewhere below the bed. Then the intravenous catheter allowed oxytocin into my vein.

My thirty-nine-year-old body seemed to have forgotten that childbirth was part of its dutiful responsibility. Gravity was not in my favor, either—I was lying in bed and expecting to push a seven-pound being through my birth canal. This, without any sensations to guide my efforts, because of an epidural. So much for mind over matter.

Where was my mother when I needed her? I had often heard her tell the story of my birth. After twelve hours of labor, my mother had walked into the delivery room and demanded the doctor, "Get this baby out, now!" The doctor had had no choice but to perform a Cesarean section and deliver me to my mother. Dr. Cove was confident Aaron was going to be born naturally. All I wanted was for the drama to be over.

As we were getting close to twelve hours of labor, Aaron finally moved down the birth canal to where his crown became visible, and the nurse was able to place a suction cup on his scalp. Finally, with the help of Dr. Cove's weight on my belly, the nurse's encouragement, and forced pushing on my part, he began to move slowly out into the ambient light.

As I was in the last minutes of labor, a nurse handed a clipboard to Sherman with some paperwork to sign.

"Why would they ask me to sign a release to administer a vaccine for Hep B to a newborn?" he asked me days later.

"Wow, he has my black hair!" Sherman said excitedly as the crown of Aaron's head began to appear. When I first saw Aaron's face, he looked calm, soft, and unmoved by the journey. Then, without shedding any tears, his life had begun.

Stories about child-rearing shared by my mother and grandmother came pouring into my consciousness. My mother, a practical woman, believed in no-fuss about anything—get on with it. Emotions only got in the way. Weeks after I was born, she returned to work. The wound on her belly had kept her home longer than she'd expected. Abuela became my primary caretaker, as both my parents worked six days a week to make ends meet and save for a house of their own—Mother as an executive secretary for a pharmaceutical company and Father as a clerk in a government office. Both made meager wages but were happy they had jobs.

Abuela's two-bedroom adobe house was my home for the first five years of my life. She taught me how to be creative and resourceful. She was a seamstress, cook, artisan, spiritual confidant, and her local church's matriarch. I often played alone in the storage room behind her kitchen, where a stack of wooden angels awaited their new threads for an upcoming procession. The smell of the paraffin Abuela used to coat petals came from the kitchen, which soon became the roses that embellished the church altar.

While Abuela sewed, I listened to stories about how she raised her seven children and all the resourceful ways she forged to keep them fed and clothed. She never let me forget about my Abuelo, an invalid, bedridden for nine years after his stroke. Memories poured into my consciousness as I began my life as a mother, and I could not forget how fortunate I was.

Breastfeeding was a hurdle as I stepped into motherhood. Aaron was slow in consenting to the "greedy love of my breasts," a description I had learned from D.W. Winnicott. Once again, I felt like my body had failed me. How could this basic instinct be so unresponsive? I thought motherhood was instinctive. It had been almost forty-eight hours since Aaron's birth, and he wouldn't take to my breast. I feared the worst for my seven-pound baby. After talking to Dr. Cove, she insisted on sending help.

"Don't be alarmed when you read 'failure to thrive' on papers they ask you to sign. That wording needs to be included for insurance reasons," Dr. Cove warned. Her words only intensified my angst. When a nurse showed up at my door, I was somewhat relieved. After asking me a few quick questions, she began to massage my breast with both hands.

"Sometimes that's all you need to get the milk going," she said, making it sound so easy. Was it me, or was it Aaron? He was not clinging or taking in the milk with enough force. Years later, I questioned this developmental step—was it part of his abnormal progression?

The nurse pressed Aaron's lips against my breast with gentle force. There was a pause that seemed longer than the seconds that passed. Then I heard a soft sucking sound and felt a tingling around my breast. What had I done wrong? It was all on me, a motherly responsibility that was now mine. I had been a mother for less than forty-eight hours. It was then I noticed self-doubt as a familiar companion. I later questioned if this rejection from the child could be what D.W. Winnicott terms fear of dependence. At that moment, all I could do was examine my ability as a mother to this dependent being.

Slowly Aaron began to take more of my natural nourishment, and I began to relax a bit. Maybe this was a natural process while our bodies synchronized to our dual rhythms, or how our lives began to merge into one.

The feeding hurdle soon receded into the past. Aaron became calm and quiet, and his serious demeanor gave him an air of innocent maturity that allowed me to feel he was developing as he should. During the checkup visit, I questioned his weight and height, and cringed when the nurse pointed out that he was below average. Dr. Cove assured me there was no need to worry. The charts, she said, were based on European examples, not on Asian and Salvadorean babies.

Looking back at those first months, signs of autism were already present. Research has contributed to the awareness of autism, and in the early 2000s, announcements began to appear in pediatricians' offices with signs that could lead to an early diagnosis.

When Aaron was seven months old, my mother, his consistent caregiver, made an observation:

"He doesn't want to sit upright. He falls over like a sack of rice," she said, half-jokingly. I didn't know what to do with this information other than keep it in my "angst box," which nagged louder as the years went on.

Later, as a toddler, Aaron showed signs of hypotonia, also known as low muscle tone. After a visit to the emergency room due to a dislocated shoulder for no apparent reason, the doctor tried to ease my angst by telling me that it was common in young children with underdeveloped muscles. As Aaron became more active, his clumsiness became more apparent; he fell regularly, but did not make a fuss. He was under-responsive to the sensory information around him and rarely cried or sought attention, unlike most toddlers do when they are connecting to the outer world. As a side note, years later as a teen, Aaron became very adept at regulating his balance. While hiking on a trail in the red hills of Sedona, Arizona, he jogged with confidence down a narrow, cactus-lined path while Sherman and I held our breaths.

Aaron was a passive baby who made few demands. We described him as easygoing. He seemed content sitting on the carpet in the living room listening to his dad play the piano and appeared oblivious to his surroundings. He focused on the music, played live, or coming from his ever-present music player, which he held close to his ear.

Aaron missed several important milestones. First, he never crawled—instead, he shaped his body like the bottom of a rocking horse and repeatedly rocked back and forth. Second, I took note of his younger girl cousins, each of whom walked before their first birthdays. Wanting to believe what I'd heard about boys developing slower than girls, I held my breath and was relieved when he took his first steps at fifteen months.

He remained unsteady on his feet until he was three or four, easily tripping over the slightest obstacle. And yet, when he stopped after twirling around while listening to music, he showed no signs of dizziness and resumed his gaze without any indication of imbalance.

Under-responsiveness to sensory stimulation was evident also in his high tolerance for pain; he seldom cried, even after a hard fall or bloody laceration.

Aaron began to speak a few words at around twelve months, and I realized he had skipped another critical milestone in language acquisition: cooing and the other sounds infants usually make during early language development. Articulation came quickly and clearly. I was surprised one day while bathing him in the kitchen sink; as water poured down his tiny body, he blurted out, "Like a diamond." The words were clear, evenly spaced, and effortless. I looked over at Sherman, puzzled for a few moments, but soon realized those were words from "Twinkle, Twinkle, Little Star," a song we often sang to him.

His vocabulary grew slowly—mostly single words in Spanish, the language my parents spoke to him. We were confident he would be trilingual, first learning Spanish and then Chinese in an immersion school. Years later, in the psychologist's office, she asked me about his use of language. I answered with pride that he had a vocabulary of about fifty words. But when the doctor asked me if he made any requests or commented on his surroundings, I could only remember a few instances: when we would walk by the toy store, and he would say balloon or musica-usica. I later realized he did not point at toys or household items, or even make simple requests with words or signs—he was repeating sounds. Repetition can be interpreted as a mild sign of echolalia.

Aunt Rose, a retired schoolteacher whom I called Tia, visited us from El Salvador to celebrate Aaron's second birthday.

"He's so serious," she said, soon after meeting Aaron. Tia had a beautiful singing voice. She and Aaron soon bonded, and she'd spend hours singing nursery rhymes in Spanish—the same ones she had sung to me when I was his age. Aaron repeated, "El Rey!" and Tia would sing it until her voice gave out. When I told his pediatrician about his repeated requests, she immediately said, "That sounds like autism." When this repetitive habit continues through childhood, it is commonly called a stim: a habitual utterance that some children (and adults) use to calm or self-regulate their nervous system.

"He looks at that book as if he's reading," Tia said. Aaron was a serene boy who seemed content with an open book in front of him; he slowly turned the pages, calmed by each one. Tia observed Aaron during her month-long visit and often commented on his serious personality. Inside, quietly, my angst was growing.

From our bedroom, we could hear the laughter and squeals that came from the backyard of a Montessori school a few houses away from ours. It was a constant reminder that it was time for Aaron to be among his peers. I finally got the courage to send him to preschool just a few months before his third birthday. The school was inviting, and the teachers were friendly.

"Why didn't you bring him sooner?" the teacher asked as she took his hand and ushered him into the play area.

A few weeks after Aaron started attending the preschool, I received a call from the head of school.

"Can you stop by my office before you pick Aaron up this afternoon?" Jim asked. My chest tightened, memories of when I was called to the principal's office returned.

I walked up the oak stairwell to Jim's office, full of angst. Each step drowned the laughter coming from the play area behind the house. I peeked into the half-opened door; Jim had his back to the door, looking out the window at the playground. I stepped over a pile of scattered wooden blocks. Next to his desk was a bookshelf of familiar books: Psychomotor Development, Language and the Mind, Dr. Montessori's Own Handbook—books I had seen on Tia's bookshelf but had never opened.

"Have a seat," he said somberly.

"I'm glad you called me. I'd like to discuss the day Aaron dislocated his elbow," I said, not giving him a chance to say a word.

"Yes, I want to hear about that, but that's not why I called you," Jim said.

"Oh?" I said as I sank slowly into a chair.

"I've been observing Aaron on the playground over the past few weeks, since the incident with his elbow." I felt the temperature in the room rise; I took off my sweater and draped it over the chair.

"He doesn't approach other children," he said, looking down at his notes. "Most of the time he plays alone in the sandbox, sifting sand through his fingers," he said quietly. I understood then why he came home with pockets full of sand. "What I'm most concerned about is that he doesn't respond to his name."

I sat unmoved.

The image I had created in my mind of Aaron surrounded by children, throwing sand on each other, laughing, playing chase—that image instantly disappeared and morphed into the sight of a lonely boy sitting in a sandbox, drowned by screams and laughter. I began a free-fall into a bottomless abyss.

"I think you should have him evaluated." Jim looked at me intently. I took a deep breath and sat in silence. "Maybe it's nothing to be alarmed about," he said in a lighter voice. Those were the words I held on to before walking out of the room. I could no longer ignore the alarms; it was time to open the "angst box."

After a week-long evaluation at the University of California, San Francisco, the call came from Dr. Lee. I already knew what she was about to tell me, yet hearing the official news left me stunned and with a dark, heavy sensation in the middle of my chest. The heaviness grew over the months, as hints of "something not right" imploded inside.

"As I suspected," she said in a slow, somber voice, "he has autism."

I don't recall anything after those words—only the heavy feeling that drew me down to my knees onto the gray carpet on our bedroom floor.

She finished by saying, "Oh, Irma! I'm so sorry." I hung up.

One Eye Open

I was born with one eye open and one closed

      in a world that does not know how to live with me

      that wants to change me, to fix me.

      The only me I have.

Some feel sorry.

      "It must be hard," they say to Mom.

      "I admire you," they say.

      What about me?

      "So sorry," they say.

      Sorry about?

Making sense of her words,

      of her tears,

      her laughter,

      her fears,

      is as impossible as making sense of their actions.

      Sometimes they hug me and tell me they love me.

      They are angry for what I can't do.

      This is the world I've been given.

A kaleidoscope world, shrieking voices that scratch my skin.

I try to understand.

They show me pictures.

They rub my arm, my legs, my back with a plastic brush.

I take their hand, they move it away.

They take my hand and push me their way.

They ask me to do what I don't understand.

I'm frustrated, I'm angry, and they don't know why.

I live among you, with you, and in you.

My inside is different, my voice is the same.

Look inside you, and you'll find me staring out.

One eye open and one eye closed.

What If

What if he was just developing slowly? What if he was confused with two languages? What if the psychologist missed something? What if he couldn't go to school? I was hyper-vigilant for words or an image that would give me a way out of this fog of unknowns. The vigilante in me caught sight of a story on a Sunday morning television show: an older woman walking down a barren road on a cold winter day, hunched over, hand in hand with her adult son. As soon as I heard the word autism, I turned the TV off. At that moment, I realized I could no longer keep the truth to myself; I needed to speak the word out loud and for someone to witness my pain. I called Desiree, a trusted friend.

In her living room, I waited, looking out her back window while she prepared tea in the kitchen. The morning fog filtered the light coming through the window as the still water on the pool slowly became visible. How I wished for the return of my capacity to look through the clear water to the bottom of a pool. Desiree tilted the porcelain teapot over my cup and handed it to me as I held my breath, not knowing where to start.

"He has autism," I blurted out, and took a sip of hot tea.

For the first time, I could say the A-word out loud. I held the cup in front of my face, looking at her, curious about her reaction. She remained calm with a slight smile on her face as if she knew something I didn't. Slowly she put her cup down on the saucer and placed her hand on my knee:

"And how are you?" she asked.

The question left me speechless. Emotions stirred within; I had no words to express how I felt—just a whirlwind of energy wanting to be released. I wished for an open field where I could see the road ahead. Where clearly marked signs guided me to my destination. Any signs. We sat in silence, tea in hand. Such a simple and unanswerable question. I took a breath and looked at her.

"I'm scared," I said. I could barely hear myself talk.

She leaned towards me and placed her hand over mine.

"What does fear look like?" she asked, her soft face gentle and curious, waiting for me to answer.

"Fear...look like?" I asked puzzled, but trusting her inquiry. I took another deep breath and closed my eyes.

"It's a big snake, yellow eyes—they're looking straight at me," I said. My body shook and my heart raced; I felt fear take over every bone in my body.

"Look straight at it!" she said with a forceful voice.

For a moment, I wavered; then a feeling of determination came over me.

"Look straight into its eyes," Desiree insisted, as if she, too, could see the snake.

After another breath, I felt the courage to close my eyes and imagine the diamond-shaped head of a giant anaconda a few inches from my face, its massive body hidden behind the triangular image. The elongated almond-shaped eye looked directly at me, and I saw my reflection. Its smooth, red tongue flicked in and out; I felt it close to me. I kept the green, scaly image in my mind for as long as I could.

My body, fully alive with fear, felt the presence of this imaginary reptile. Minutes passed, and then something happened: I felt the snake become part of me. It was no longer inside my mind. Now it was entirely in my body.

When I left Desiree's home and stepped out into the late morning, I felt the coolness of the air on my forearms and heard birds and the gardener blowing leaves from the driveway into the gully.

My father had told me a story about walking alone in the dense, tropical forest close to his home as a young boy. Darkness fell before he could return home, so he prepared a campsite to spend the night in the wilderness. He woke up to a slimy sensation under his neck. From the corner of his eye, he could see the leaves tremble around him. He felt the sensual body of a black snake slowly moving into the darkness. When he recounted this story, he said he was sure the snake had kept vigil all night for him and left when she knew he was safe. I'm not sure how much of that story was true, but he turned it into a lesson for me.

Snakes have a way of showing up in my life. When I was a young girl, I frequented our local church with my abuela. At the entrance stood a statue of the Virgin Mary. She had one foot resting on a globe and the other flattening a snake's head. Then, as we entered, Abuela touched Virgin Mary's feet, crossed her forehead, and ended with a reverential kiss of her thumb. For years I followed her, doing the same ritual, not knowing the meaning behind the act. The snake is a powerful symbol of transformation, and it appeared again, serving to walk me gently and firmly from fear to courage.

I have to be honest; I didn't know that I had been transformed that morning. Only twenty-some years later could I begin to understand what had happened to me. I left Desiree's home a different person, trusting I was being guided and ready to move through the dense fog without the need to know what was in front of me.

The White Binder

Dr. Lee was candid about her lack of knowledge about autism. After all, in 1997, it was not as familiar a diagnosis as it is today, in 2022.

"I have something that may help you," she said, and handed me a two-inch binder full of articles and hand-written notes.

It came from Charlotte, a mother who lived just a few miles from our home. She was a mother to two sons with autism. Dr. Lee warned about the lack of medical treatment and reminded me there was no cure. The binder gave me not only a starting point, but also a credible resource from a caring mother who had gone through the painful journey herself.

"Focus on communication," she said as I was ready to leave her office. "It's a core deficit and will help him navigate the world."

Without fully realizing the value of this work of love from a mother, I stacked the binder on top of unread books about autism. At that time, I wasn't ready to dive into it. The shock of the diagnosis was still very present, and the experience with Desiree had not fully landed for me. I had used every ounce of confidence I had to say the A-word, as many referred to autism in those days.

It was Sherman who gave me the ultimatum I needed to move forward. His words woke me up to the reality we were both facing.

"If you don't do something about Aaron, I will leave the company and do it myself," he said one morning, with a determined look I had not seen before.

"I don't know where to start," I said, shaking with fear.

"The window of opportunity for him to learn is closing. We have to do something!" he said in an unwavering voice.

At that moment, I relinquished the fear and stepped into the unknown. Aaron was almost four years old, and time was not in his favor. I was constantly reminded of this critical period of brain development and we needed to act quickly if he was to have a chance to learn skills that would allow him to become a functional adult.

One morning, when the house was quiet—Sherman had left for the office and Aaron was out at the park with my mother—I took the white binder, took a deep breath, and opened it to the first page.

I imagined Charlotte carefully arranging the pages inside the binder, imagining the mother that would one day use it as a trail guide for the journey ahead. Taped on blue-lined paper were articles—some from Reader's Digest, others from Developmental Psychology, and a clipping from an Ann Lander's column. It was a goldmine: phone numbers, names of doctors, therapists, teachers, and parents who probably guided her. Next to each name was a brief synopsis of the value or lack thereof. Hand-written notes guided me through the pages. "Keep eye on wallet" was penciled in next to the name of a physician with a San Francisco address. Further down the page, "Don't expect a call right away. Keep trying." Arrows pointed to several names. Circled in red on a note: good therapist, not-so-good bedside manner. A well-known doctor's name was underlined with a note: They call him a quack but he has important information.

She cited books by Catherine Maurice, a mother with two children on the spectrum; Donna Williams, a young woman with autism; and Temple Grandin, an engineer who was becoming well known for designing a humane way to treat livestock. The white binder was full of information. I began to relax as I discerned the next step through the fog of uncertainty. More importantly, the binder gave me a place from which to start my own discovery process—guidance I had expected to find inside the psychologists' reports after week-long evaluations. Instead, what we had heard was, "Have a glass of wine, take a warm bath, and good luck. Oh, and when he's ready, call the school district and start the IEP process." I had no idea what an IEP was and why the school district would help me with a medical condition.

A side note: It took determined parents years to change state laws. Now, in 2022, forty-six states require insurance companies to pay for specific therapeutic treatments for autism.

Each note in the binder was a marker leading me to the next step, then to the next signpost that, just maybe, would help me move ahead. Questions began to appear and in them would be the next one, like crumbs leading me somewhere. And I didn't need to know where that was. The fog in my mind began to lift as I took one step at a time. The truth became clear: Aaron would not develop like a neurotypical child. So, I looked for a path away from a precipice.

It all seemed so much bigger than me. I hadn't realized how small and incapable I took myself to be. That belief was hidden under a thin cloud of invincibility and the belief that I could fix anything. I know it sounds contradictory. I later learned I was following a pattern that helped me deal with life's demands and, by doing so, I was not accessing the truth and core of my true nature, which is what I needed most to guide me on this path.

Now, a mother with more experience and knowledge than me was holding my hand. I had never met Charlotte; we began a conversation about our sons through the binder. I was ready to continue the journey, so I took the next step on an unmarked path called autism.

The Boy in the Room

"Popular behavioral therapist" was written on a note card. What was a behavioral therapist? How could a child so young be ready for therapy? I picked up the phone, paused for a moment, then dialed the number.

I left a message on her voice mail, expecting a response in a few days. A month or so later the therapist called back, asking for a video recording of Aaron before she would schedule a visit.

I tried to capture moments that showed his sweetness: sitting in the playroom looking like a wise Buddha, staring out the window as he strummed his thumb against his right cheek. I caught him as he listened to Sherman playing Beethoven's sonatas as he twirled around in the living room like a Sufi dancer. I was hoping to hear comments about his gift as a dancer. Sherman captured a moment when I called his name while he was on the kitchen table, being spoon-fed by his abuela.

"Aaron, look at Mama," I said joyfully; there was no response.

"Look at Mama," his abuela repeated. When he didn't respond, she took his face with both hands and moved it towards me. He didn't object to the manipulation and stared out into space.

"Mom, please!" I shouted at her.

"But he doesn't understand you," she shouted back. The tension between us began to escalate. We began to talk less and less. The stress brought about the awareness that Aaron had an incurable syndrome—it was about to consume us all. Mother didn't want to talk about the specifics of how to deal with the unresponsiveness she was seeing in Aaron. Underneath, I felt like there must have been some way I could have prevented this. My Catholic upbringing was surfacing, and guilt became overwhelming.

"Let's just leave it as it is. We can deal with it later," Sherman said, and he put away the video camera.

Six months later, when Dianne, an ABA (Applied Behavior Analysis) therapist, finally showed up to assess Aaron, we were ready and eager to see what therapy was all about. She was in demand at that time, and I was grateful to finally get her on the schedule. I was eager to learn from her interaction with Aaron.

She walked straight to Aaron's room and sat at the child-sized table, organizing her writing pad and three plastic blocks while she waited for me to bring Aaron in. She placed red, blue, and yellow blocks in front of Aaron and waited. She remained silent. Aaron sat in the chair, dangling a set of keys in front of his face. After a few seconds, she scribbled some notes on her yellow pad.

"Give me yellow," she said without emotion. Aaron continued to flick his keys with his fingers. From where I stood, he seemed to be trying to ignore the therapist. What I learned later was that he was coping with an overload of sensory stimulation. He found a stim, or self-stimulatory behavior that helped him cope with the demands he was facing.

"Aaron!" she said calmly but firmly. Aaron continued to stim. The light passed through his fingers when he moved them, creating a visual image that must have been calming for him. After a few seconds, she wrote a long string of notes on her notepad before moving a yellow block closer to Aaron.

"Give me yellow," she said in the same flat tone of voice. Aaron continued to stim without changing his gaze. She waited, scribbled some more, and moved the yellow block even closer to the edge of the table.

"Aaron…give me yellow," she asked for the third time. Aaron didn't move. I wondered what she was scribbling on the yellow pad. This interaction continued for several minutes. When that didn't get Aaron's attention, she used a toy car, miniature dolls, and different-sized blocks, all without a response.

After thirty minutes filled with a litany of requests, she stopped and began writing longer notes on her pad. I stood outside, looking into the room through a one-way mirror that permitted me to observe without interrupting his sessions. Without rising from his chair, Aaron continued to look at his fingers in front of his face. "He's so patient," I thought. Just months before, he was unable to sit for any period of time, roaming around the room as his teacher, Patty called him over and over back to the chair. In searching for signs of progress, I saw a new skill: waiting.

"I'll write the report and send it to you within the next month," she said. "I don't have a spot available for him at this time, but you can use the report to get someone else to work with him. It should give them an idea of where he is," she finished quickly, leaving no room for me to ask any questions. She gathered her notes and headed towards the door.

"Oh, I almost forgot," she said as she pulled out a video from her satchel. It was the introductory tape she had requested as a "virtual interview." "The music in the background was lovely," she said, and closed the door behind her.

After months of waiting for a visit from the acclaimed therapist, I was disappointed. Is this what we're in for? There must be other people who saw Aaron as a person—not something that needed fixing. Or maybe I just didn't know enough about autism.

My gut feeling was that there must be another way. I couldn't get myself behind the popular beliefs I kept reading about.

Relieved by the opening Dianne gave me to find another therapist, I continued my search. I never called her again. She had ignored the boy in the room. I wondered if I was doing the same.

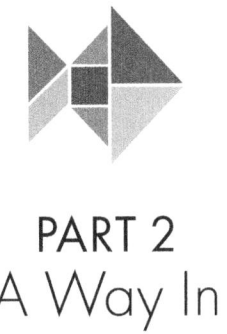

PART 2
A Way In

"The connections made by good teachers are
held not in their methods but in their hearts."

—*The Courage to Teach*,
Parker J. Palmer

Hope

"He-llooo A a a r o o n," Patty said in a slow, soprano tone as she entered his playroom.

Aaron sat in his usual place on the carpeted floor, his back to the door, bottom resting between his chubby thighs like a yogi in a meditative pose, undisturbed by the thump that followed when she released two canvas bags onto the floor. His room was bright, with two large windows that let the morning light in. The corner room looked out on a century-old redwood tree on one side and an evergreen silk tree on the other. At night the light from the streetlamp didn't seem to bother Aaron, but truly, there wasn't much that bothered him.

Hope was palpable, though far away. Inside the white binder, Patty's name was written, along with a note: May not answer but keep trying.

She was cheerful and undisturbed by Aaron's lack of response. I, on the other hand, was just getting used to the void left by the silence. He began to talk around the age of two. By the time Patty began to work with Aaron, around the age of four, he seldom said a word. The loss of words began with stuttering when saying the names of his favorite Sesame Street characters. Gradually, he spoke less and less until he was left with the occasional Big Bird or Barney. Maybe, just maybe, the words would slowly come back. I was willing to wait. Patty brought hope into our home.

Next to the east-facing window was a small table and two chairs just the right size for Aaron, which I had bought at a specialty store with the hope that someday he would draw or paint with a friend or two. But he preferred to sit on the floor and pushed away anything that resembled a crayon, pencil, or any other drawing instrument. Patty re-arranged the table, placing it against the corner of the room so Aaron was corralled by her long legs.

"How are you today?" she asked as she walked around the room arranging cards, books, and puzzles on the small tabletop. She continued to talk, without expecting an answer from Aaron.

"I love that tie-dye shirt you are wearing," she said.

"That cookie looks yummy; are you going to finish it?" She pointed to the half-eaten cookie on the table.

Aaron remained silent, listening to the muffled sounds coming from a set of plastic keys he held next to his ear and tapped in a quick motion, as if there was a message far away meant just for him.

Patty was a tall woman, handsome, with short, coiffed, blond hair and fair skin, which would turn red at the slightest embarrassing thought. I was surprised to hear a voice after the first ring.

"I only work on weekends," she said in a firm voice. She left little room for negotiation.

"Is there a church close to your house? Catholic, I mean," she asked. I was ready to accommodate her wish. I imagined she and my mother walking together across the street to St. Matthew's for early-morning Mass.

"Almost right across the street. You can even walk there," I said.

"No, I'll come after Mass," she said. A few weeks later, we began a relationship that has lasted for years.

"Now that I'm a widow, I can focus my time on these kids," she said. "I miss being in the classroom, but, well…" she said. I knew then we'd found the right person. She soon became part of our family.

During the week Patty worked at an autism clinic. She interviewed parents with more than one autistic child. Her experience and connections proved helpful; soon we had young interns working with her and engaging Aaron for two hours at a time. I'll never forget the first time she visited us. It was torture for me.

"Aaron, come sit with me," she said as she tapped on the chair next to her.

Aaron didn't move from the corner of the room. His long, black hair hid the fact that his eyes were fixed on the carpet, as he totally focused on the music from his tape player. After the third or fourth request, she took his hand and walked with him to the table where they sat next to each other. Immediately, Aaron got up.

"You need to sit in the chair," she said in a melodic voice and once again gently took his hand, held his thighs down, and insisted he sit down again.

"Oops, where are you going?" she asked, and brought him back again and again and again. This went on for what felt like forever but it was only about half an hour. I looked on through the one-way mirror.

"He needs to be table-ready. Otherwise, he will never make it in school," she said to me as she left the room. My angst must have been evident.

"Don't worry. He'll learn. We'll continue doing this until he sits down without any prompts." She sounded sure of herself, and it gave me confidence that she knew what she was doing. This was all new to me, and all I could do was trust. But inside, my heart was breaking.

After the third day of following the drill of getting up and coming back to the chair, Aaron finally stayed sitting for a few seconds—long enough to get praise from Patty.

"Good sitting in the chair!" she said. Then he got his reward. "Now you can go get a hug from Mama," she said, and he ran over to me for comfort.

Every thirty seconds he was allowed to get up and get his "reward hug." Then back to the chair. She increased the time between hugs to one, two, three, and then four minutes. Over time his rewards were prolonged until books, cards, and toys became interesting to him.

"Aaron, I need a break!" she'd say, and set the timer on his desk. Aaron was becoming more and more interested in the blocks and books Patty brought each week, and there was a time when he wanted to continue past the two-hour time limit. The timer became an important tool; it gave Aaron an idea of how long he needed to wait, a skill that needs to be explicitly taught to those with autism. Not knowing what to expect next can be excruciating. I learned this from Sherman who, after he reflected on the evaluation results for Aaron, was certain he, too, was autistic, on the other side of the spectrum.

Patty had a dramatic way of reading—she added sound effects and body movements. She turned herself into a bear and pretended to move over mountains or made sounds of a train coming down the track when she read Thomas the Tank Engine. Aaron began to show interest in books by Dr. Seuss and the most traditional nursery rhymes. Patty read them over and over again until she could no longer bear the repetition herself.

Patty introduced him to nouns and verbs written on flash cards with images of zoo animals, children riding bikes, and breakfast and lunch foods. With enthusiasm, she'd hold up a card in front of his face and label it for him, giving it meaning. Then came the test. She placed two cards in front of him and in a monotone voice:

"Give me bear," she said, and held out her hand. He hesitated for a moment and then handed her the card with a brown grizzly bear.

"Excellent, Aaron!" she said, giving him effusive praise.

"Give me elephant," she continued.

"Good!" Praise became his reward, but only after he looked up at her.

This exercise became one of his favorite activities while in the room with Patty. Soon he could recognize most of the three hundred pictures in the box. The two hours in the playroom with Patty were like play. As time passed and Aaron asked for more focused interaction, she recruited others to engage with him. Soon there were three people in the room throughout the day. Each person was trained and mentored by Patty on how to best engage Aaron. This can be a very expensive process.

A note to all parents: laws have been adopted that provide the intensive support required by people with autism. Parent support groups are a great way to learn and keep up to date with the new laws and regulations. During the early years after Aaron's diagnosis, support groups helped us find information that was not readily accessible.

Gradually, Aaron began to engage more with Sherman and me. Patty became a resource for us and always highlighted the slightest signs that opened opportunities for interaction. Books about autism began to make sense—now we could be more confident in trying new approaches to engage with our son. Slowly, Aaron began to emerge from his world, giving us hope.

There were many more teachers that came into our home and supported Aaron through his school years; some are still in our lives and have left lasting and heartfelt memories. One woman who touched us and embodied the love that others had shared with Aaron was Danielle. She devoted many weekends to our home during her undergraduate years. When it was time for her to continue her graduate studies in clinical psychology, she told us with tears in her eyes that she was moving to San Diego.

"But I will be coming to the Bay Area to visit my family, and of course I'll come to see Aaron," she said with a smile that parted her tears.

There was a calm and joyful energy when she entered Aaron's playroom. Music and laughter came through the closed door that separated Aaron's bedroom from the playroom. Her time with him was so natural—just two people enjoying each other's company. Looking back, her enthusiasm and smile were possibly more powerful than the therapy skills he was learning from the academics. Danielle taught Aaron that people could be fun, and he didn't need to do anything to earn their love. He learned to trust her and developed a personal connection that seemed joyful and engaging. During their time together they danced, laughed, and read books, over and over.

After Danielle moved to San Diego, she continued to visit Aaron. She spent more time at the airport than in Aaron's playroom. She wove in stories of good times with friends—attempts to make me feel less guilty for her long commute. I'm certain Aaron's current love of books and his self-taught reading skills started back when he and Danielle sat on the blue mat in his playroom reading Chicka Chicka Boom Boom. She read that story many times, always relishing Aaron's unashamed joy. After the end of each book, she would say with a smile, "The end." That was his cue to pick up the next book and hand it over.

"Hiiiii! Aaaaaron!" She'd drop down to her knee when she saw Aaron at the front door. Every word had energy and emotion attached to it. She took Aaron's small hand in hers and they walked into his playroom. For two hours they were engaged, the door closed, the same three books and music from a small boom box their only companions. I remember our last conversation on the way to the United terminal, where I dropped her off.

"What has kept you coming back to see Aaron?" I asked her.

"I guess the obvious answer is love, for you and for him. He crawled into my heart. I was hooked!" she said with a smile that still brings tears to my eyes.

Many teachers have come into our home. They continue living their lives—getting married, raising their own children, losing loved ones, and experiencing the pains and joys of life. What they have left behind is the hope that love does not need words.

Play: Children's Work

Gloria, an energetic occupational therapist (OT), opened the door to the charming, one-story house in the midst of a suburban neighborhood. It was a welcomed change from the white-washed clinics we were used to visiting. Toys were piled in large bins in the corners of every room. Small, well-worn, child-sized tables were scattered around, but mostly the rooms were empty of furniture. It was clear this was a place where kids came to play. In the background, I heard muffled playground sounds. I listened carefully to Gloria as she explained the magic that took place in the small house.

"We recruit expert players from the school next door. They should be here any minute. That's when this place comes alive," she said with a big smile. I began to understand the message on a poster at the entrance of the clinic: Play is children's work.

Aaron's therapy sessions were not what I had imagined. He was six years old when he began a version of Integrated Play Therapy with expert players at least two years older than he. The boys came into the room, gathered blocks, cars, and a few rag dolls and sat next to Aaron on the floor. He looked like a typical child sitting with his peers as they pushed trucks and cars across the floor. Gloria called this parallel play, the first step for introducing play to children with autism.

"Vroooooom," Peter said, and guided a wooden block up Aaron's back as he sat, unmoved by the activity in the room.

"Look, Aaron, it's going up a hill," the boy said.

Peter wasn't bothered by Aaron's ambivalence and went on playing with Tom, the other expert player in the room. Tom and Peter moved close to Aaron and engaged him when they saw an opportunity. Aaron's participation was in his willingness to stay within close proximity to the other boys and be part of the action going on around him.

This therapy is based on work done by Dr. Pamela Wolfberg, who promoted play as a critical part of socialization. Her premise was based on research that showed that autistic children can engage in play with neurotypical peers while supported in mutually enjoyed experiences. The expert players "taught" their autistic peers by engaging in natural play activities and responding to natural cues. They played without a goal but with perceptive eyes and awareness of what was going on around them. This was a rich teaching experience for all the children involved.

Play addresses the sensory needs of every child. I was slowly learning that Aaron's system was out of sync and in need of more direct and consistent engagement in natural activities. Over the years I've learned to connect with my own sensations through meditation and body awareness. I first became aware of how unconformable being inside my body could be after a yoga class that was followed by a short meditation. While I was dying inside, I opened my eyes to see how everyone else was doing. Others seemed totally at ease, sitting with their legs crossed, arms resting on their laps. Inside my body I felt as if a swarm of ants was moving through my veins. Ten minutes felt like hours. I could only imagine the discomfort Aaron must have felt when his sensory system was active and he could not verbalize his discomfort. He developed his own self-regulation strategies that seemed abnormal to those who didn't understand him.

Aaron skipped some of the developmental steps that are part of learning balance and movement. Crawling was never part of his development. He went straight to walking. With the guidance of an occupational therapist, he was learning how to regulate his system and catch up on the gaps.

In the clinic he joined others in one of his favorite activities—twirling inside a spandex swing. The joy on his face was undeniable. Peter took advantage of the visible excitement.

"Swinging, swinging, swinging Aaron, gently down the stream," he sang to the tune of "Row, Row, Row Your Boat." They both smiled in a mutual enjoyment that was part of this therapeutic model that was crucial for Aaron's development. I was overjoyed to see him playing—playing like a typical child.

The role of an occupational therapist was becoming clear to me. In the clinic, through play and interaction, a major deficit was being addressed: sensory processing. Dr. A. Jean Ayres explained the role of the occupational therapist in autism treatment and linked sensory imbalance (hyper or hyposensitivity) to unusual interests or behaviors. Aaron's obsessions began to make sense and it became clear why bells, chimes, twirling around the room, running sand through his fingers, and staring at light passing through the blinds engaged him in such a hypnotic way. He was self-regulating his system. His behavior didn't need to be changed, but observed and understood.

Mirroring

Her name was written on the first page of the white binder next to this note, which caught my interest: Kind woman, mother who has much to share. It was Marcia who first introduced me to the work of Barry and Mariah Kaufman, parents who recovered their eighteen-month-old son Raun from autism. When they were told by medical professionals that there was nothing they could do to treat their autistic son, they took it upon themselves to help him. This led them to develop a method that later turned into a program called Son-Rise. I was moved by their defiance and became curious about the approach the Kaufmans used with Raun. When Marcia came to our home, I felt her kindness and willingness to share what she knew.

"Can I meet Aaron?" she asked as soon as she entered our home—even before we had a chance to introduce ourselves.

"I'll bring him down," I said. A few moments later I walked into the den, holding Aaron in my arms. He was four at the time and still small enough for me to carry him.

"Does he walk?" she asked, and I promptly placed him down on the floor. Marcia sat on the floor next to him.

"Hi, Aaron, my name is Marcia," she said, looking to meet his eyes, but he continued to look at the book he was carrying.

"I like Dr. Seuss, too," she said. He continued to look away. There was silence for a long time; uncomfortable for me, but she seemed at ease in the space between the three of us.

"I'm going to talk to your mom now. It was nice meeting you," she said as she got up off the floor. Aaron sat looking at the book.

We talked about her background in education and a bit about her family life. She took a book from her satchel and handed it to me.

"It's worth reading," she said.

She was right, and after reading the book Son-Rise by Barry Neil Kaufman, I enrolled in a week-long introductory program at The Options Institute. The institute was located in the Berkshires atop a bluff overlooking a wide-open river valley, with rolling hills in the background and a dense forest in the foreground. Cabins and spacious, rustic meeting rooms were scattered throughout the one-hundred-acre grounds. Trails and lakes, which allowed space for reflection and contemplation, added to the expansive beauty of the retreat center. My intention was to find a treatment that would bring Aaron back from his autistic tendencies. I was surprised when I realized that the week-long retreat was all about my own mindset and beliefs, which had influenced my parenting biases. I was guided by a coach, who led me to examine the automatic coping strategies that were part of the way I showed up as a parent of an atypical child. Many years later, as I began to understand my personality patterns, I realized I was using these strategies and beliefs in interactions with others as well. At that time in my life, this was the only way I could handle the pain caused by the sudden realization that my son was not the child I expected him to be.

What I learned at the Institute changed my relationship with Aaron. It propelled me on a journey that had begun in my late teens as a curious young artist.

I will never forget the life drawing class, in front of a naked male model, where I asked myself the question: who is observing me?

As I struggled to get the right dimensions of the model on my sketch pad, I realized there was an inner voice censoring each mark I made on the paper, marks prompted every time I gazed self-consciously at the model's naked body. Who was observing my actions and my emotions? I felt a sense of shame; where was it coming from? Everyone around the room was seriously moving their gaze between the paper and the model. I kept fighting with the commotion in my mind, while maintaining movement of the charcoal pencil around the white space.

Over the years, I've become closer to that observer—the one that observes how beliefs guide my behavior. This reflective capacity has led me towards becoming a more transparent inquirer into my own child's atypical behaviors. It's invited curiosity about what is going on inside of him and me.

The basic premise of the Son-Rise program was to bring light to the power of an honest and open relationship with my son—one that allowed me to accept him and meet him where he was.

The cornerstone of the Son-Rise program was the examination of our own beliefs. Sherman was hesitant; he was convinced that the methods based on applied behavior analysis (ABA) were the right treatment models. This conflict between the ways we wanted to parent Aaron created tension in our marriage.

I kept a focus on giving the Son-Rise method a try and placed our names on a six-month waiting list. The plan was for Patty, my sister-in-law Pat, Sherman, Aaron, and me to engage in a week-long program in the Berkshires.

Sherman went along with the plan until the evening before we were scheduled to leave for the Institute. As I was packing, I heard footsteps downstairs moving from one side of the dining room to the other. As I turned on the lights, there was Sherman, pacing the room in the dark.

"Is everything Okay?" I asked.

"I can't go," Sherman said in a determined voice.

"What!" I said, angry and confused.

"Our flight is tomorrow morning! Why are you telling me this now?" I tried to stay calm.

"I don't know how talking about our feelings will help Aaron. How is this going to fix him?" he said in an angry voice. "We need to enroll him in an ABA program, not spend money on talk therapy," he said.

At that moment, all I was faced with was a choice between my marriage and my son.

"I'm going to bed. Let's talk about this tomorrow," I said.

The next morning, Mother came over early to prepare Aaron's suitcase for his first cross-country trip: Winnie the Pooh book, Raffi cassette tape, word cards box, red-checkered flannel shirt and footed pajamas she had bought for the trip. By then, Aaron was almost five.

"I heard it's cold in Massachusetts," she said before leaving. "Don't forget to take his hat," she uttered in a quiet voice.

"Sí, Mama," I said.

I touched her shoulder; she quickly turned without looking at me, and picked up her coat, which was lying on a chair. Mother had a way of disguising her emotions.

"Call us when you get there," she said. I followed her as she walked out the door. "I hope they can help him." Her voice trailed away as she closed the car door. We rarely talked about autism or how it was affecting Aaron, never mind the impact it was having on our family. She seldom asked questions. As she drove away, I wished she could share her sadness with me. What I really wanted was to share mine and the conflict surfacing between Sherman and me.

Sherman came downstairs, suitcase in one hand and airline tickets, maps, and printed directions to the Institute in the other.

"I'm going…I'll give it a try," he said. For the first time, I felt a distant hopefulness. That's all I could manage.

I breathed a sigh of relief. The grogginess from a sleepless night disappeared.

Late fall in the Berkshires is breathtaking. Traces of golden foliage were still visible on the branches. A sprawling campus overlooked a lush forest of greens with infrequent shades of orange and amber. Sheffield, Massachusetts, was a small town, away from the frenzy of a large city. It was time for our whole family to embrace Aaron in this adventure. Aunt Pat was eager to learn more about personal engagement and to connect with Aaron in a more intimate way. She had a good mentor in Patty; it was now time to go deeper. Patty was more familiar with the traditional ABA methods, with a touch of love and relationship-building techniques she had brought back from the years when she'd taught young children in the public school. Yet she was hesitant about this relationship approach to engagement.

"We're going to confuse him," Patty said, when I first told her about the institute.

"This is more about us than about him," I'd said to her.

"I will do this for Aaron, but know that I'm not totally supportive of this," she'd said. "Where's the data?" she'd asked. Reluctantly, she joined us for the program.

Part of the intensive, week-long program was focused on Aaron, from morning to evening. Before breakfast, a young man came to the cabin, gently took Aaron by the hand and walked with him to a wide-open room in an adjacent building. Throughout the day, young, energetic facilitators filled with optimism engaged with Aaron inside the room, each taking a two-hour shift. A one-way mirror gave us a front-row view of the activity in the room. After dinner, another young person brought him back to the cabin, where we unwound from the long day of activity.

The facilitators had one objective: follow Aaron through the day and mirror his slightest movements. When Aaron turned around and around, the facilitator did the same. When he walked towards the door and turned the knob, the facilitator mimicked his hand turning the knob. At first, Aaron's actions were centered on going towards the door; then he settled into more engagement with his room partners.

What began to happen inside that room after a few days was subtle and unexpected: Aaron began to pay attention to the young men and women with whom he was sharing space. The facilitators began to respond to the slightest communication intent, each present to what was needed in the moment. They moved with Aaron, allowing him to give them permission to enter his world.

While Aaron was in the room, Sherman, Patty, Pat, and I were going through an inquiry process with individual coaches and in groups. This exchange was meant to look at the beliefs we each had around autism, teaching, and engaging with Aaron.

Over the years that followed, we continued the practice of following Aaron's lead. Slowly my relationship with Aaron began to mature. It was an excruciating process, but one that changed us both. This way of being with a child was so different from what I had learned growing up: the parents and adults offered knowledge and lessons, while the child had nothing to give back but obedience.

As we ended this week of intense introspection, the group of parents who had come to learn how to change their children sat in a circle, ready to share their perspectives of the week. We sat on the floor in a large meeting room, surrounded by windows overlooking a dense grove of aspen trees, notebooks in hand. The morning started with a request from the facilitator: she asked us to take as much time as we needed and write a letter to our son or daughter, one that I would read to Aaron twenty years later. When everyone was finished, the facilitator stood in the middle of the room.

"Who would like to share what they wrote to their child?" she asked. Slowly, hands began to rise. After I read my letter to the group and we were ready to leave, a grandmother came and stood before me, grabbing my shoulders with her two hands.

"Do you really think your son's autism is a blessing?" she asked.

I stood frozen for a moment as I looked into her blue eyes, her white hair touched by the sunlight pouring through the window behind her.

"Yes, he is a blessing," I answered, and at that moment, something changed within me that has guided me through his life.

I removed the burden of change from Aaron. Everything I had learned up to that time was focused on changing his behavior, changing who he was. I had never questioned the behavior of the teachers or therapists, yet I had known in my gut something was incongruent. I just hadn't known what to do with that awareness.

The experience at the Options Institute opened many more questions: How does our interior well-being impact Aaron? How was I getting in my own way? What if I joined his world? How would that change him? How would it change me? How would it change our family?

Many years later, as I entered the field of education, these questions re-emerged and I was guided by work that focused on the foundational principle expressed by Parker J. Palmer: relational trust is built on movements of the human heart.

Outside World

We returned from the Berkshires with new optimism. The playroom was where I began to observe changes in Aaron. The room became a replica of the one at the Options Institute, where Aaron coexisted with alternating facilitators throughout the ten-hour days. Toys were kept within his view but out of reach. The design of the room was meant to promote interaction and initiation. All signs of self-expression would be attended. Intentions were as important as goals—a way of finding new doorways into his world. A sound, a movement of his finger, a gaze towards a toy, each was an invitation for engagement. Self-aware companions would respond by engaging Aaron and prompting another circle of communication. What seemed like inactive stares between Aaron and his partner were signs of engagement. After a day of uninterrupted interplay, the house would finally become quiet and we could enjoy some family time. The intensity of engagement was purposeful and was intended to create a personal bond with Aaron by mirroring his every action and then responding to his slightest communicative intent. If he scratched his nose, his friend would do the same; if he twirled, jumped, or just looked at his fingers, his partner would follow.

In his book The Child, the Family, and the Outside World, D.W. Winnicott points out that for a neurotypical four-year-old, it is legitimate for his inner world to be inside as well as outside. We enter into the child's inner world when we interact with them through play. We don't say children don't fly; we pick them up and fly them around the room. For reasons that continue to be the subject of many studies, autistic children don't engage in imaginative play and tend to express themselves in pragmatic ways. An autistic individual can be seen as an extreme introvert, living in his own world. Of the many interventions I read about, those that felt promising were based on increasing Aaron's curiosity about the outside world by engaging with him in activities he himself initiated, unlike therapies which were based on teacher-driven tasks. This way of interaction enabled us to become part of Aaron's world, as we joined him in jumping, twirling, looking out the window, or just sitting in silence.

Many birthday presents remained unopened, neatly stacked in the closet ready for the day when he may be interested in trucks, Legos, blocks, or dolls. His only play toys were those that made high-pitched sounds, with the exception of his red plastic tricycle. He'd turn it upside down and spin the black wheel over and over, observing it with interest. When it fully stopped, he'd gently give it another tap and gaze as it spun around, again and again.

I became more aware of how much I anticipated his needs and realized the importance of slowing down, noticing my own internal reactions, and making time and space for Aaron to express his own wants and needs, at his pace. Slowly I began to observe and listen from a different place, where my focus wasn't on fixing him. I became curious about this little being in front of me.

We covered the floor of his playroom with a thickly padded mat, mostly for the adult facilitator who knelt or sat close to him and interacted face to face. Up on the shelves were books, a small keyboard, and a music player. Clearly within sight was his favorite toy, a red plastic car that, when the fender was touched, made a loud, blaring sound. I remembered Dr. Lee's one and only piece of advice: focus on communication. This is what we learned at the Institute— the first step was to create a safe space for him to communicate and want to be with us. We made no demands or requests. I began to see the world through his eyes, as did the others who signed up to spend time with him in the room.

This was a different approach from the one we had seen through ABA therapy, where the focus of the interaction was to teach skills. The secret to engagement was in creating trust in the relationship. I recruited individuals who believed in this approach and introduced them to what we had learned at the Institute.

This way of interacting with children was not new; it had been introduced in the 1970s by Dr. Stanley Greenspan and it became known as the Floortime Approach. He advocated that emotional experiences drive communication and thinking.

Over time, we began to see a change in Aaron and a desire to engage and be with those who joined him in the playroom. Patty recruited and mentored young men and women who had an interest in learning about autism from the clinic where she worked. As the months progressed, the facilitators came to develop their own personal connection with Aaron, taking turns reading, dancing, and following his lead. At times I peered inside the room through the one-way mirror; their interaction seemed like play and he was engaged with another person! Each responded naturally to Aaron's cues, which motivated him to become more and more connected to his partner. Part of their engagement was giving him choices and taking turns reinforcing his attempts with natural rewards, like reading and singing his favorite songs.

After a few months of Floortime activities, Aaron began to interact more with others. My sister-in-law, Pat, became a regular in the playroom. They developed a close relationship, which has lasted through the years. She joined what we called the A-team, mentored by Patty.

There are benefits to the ABA and discrete-trial approaches. They are meant to teach practical skills like following directions and labeling items—prerequisites for language acquisition.

"This is the entrance exam to kindergarten," Patty would remind me. She continued to use this teacher-driven approach while others used the Floortime model.

ABA was instrumental in teaching Aaron toileting skills, one of the most valuable lessons in his early years. Patty outlined a plan that began a week-long intensive training. With a portable toilet placed conveniently inside his playroom, while juice and his favorite music toys were kept close by his side, teachers took two-hour shifts focusing on this one skill. Each drop of urine in the plastic toilet earned him access to his music toy.

These skills were preparing Aaron for what I wanted most for him—to be in a school with other children and run on the playground and play rough-and-tumble games with other boys. I saw the long hours in the room as necessary if he were to one day attend a school that wasn't labeled special.

Our home became like a clinic, with people in and out throughout the day. We were rarely alone. We accepted this lack of privacy as part of Aaron's preparation for the larger world. Patty's teaching and consistent drills began to pay off. Aaron was able to sit for a prolonged period of time and began to learn. The drills became a part of their interaction:

"Show me cookie," she'd say, and hold out her hand. "Yay, Aaron, yes, that's a cookie," she'd respond with enthusiasm.

"Show me slide," she'd say, and place three new cards on the table. She only gave positive praise and was consistent in not showing disappointment in a wrong answer.

"Try again," she'd say with a smile, and move the correct card closer to him. "That's the slide," she'd say as she guided his hand towards the correct card.

Then there were the action cards. Those were the most challenging for Aaron.

"Show me the girl on the swing," she'd instruct, and wait as he looked carefully at the girls on the cards, one holding a ball, one kicking a ball, and another sitting on a swing.

"That's it! Yes, the girl is swinging!" She'd applaud.

Two hours would pass, and Aaron seemed eager to continue. Patty was intrigued by his perseverance, and she continued to challenge him. Her next task was teaching him how to write.

She placed a blank sheet of paper in front of Aaron and handed him a crayon. He took the crayon and threw it into an empty trash can. He then took it out and threw it back in, over and over, more interested in the sound it made than the blank piece of paper on the desk.

"Okay, Aaron, time to do some writing," she said as she retrieved the crayon out of the trash can.

"Let's draw a line. Then you can play with the red car," she said as she placed the crayon in Aaron's palm, cupped her hand around his and traced a line between two dots.

"Well done, you've made a line," she said as she handed Aaron the red car. His frown quickly turned into a big smile.

When it was time to transition from home to the neighborhood school, I began to search for what would continue to stretch Aaron's world and give him social experiences with children his age.

Everyone used the word special to identify Aaron and his classroom, teachers, and therapists. The word replaced the once-common labels of handicapped or disabled. I began to visit special schools, all within driving distance from our home.

"Don't worry about transportation," the director said as she handed me the list of special schools. "He will be picked up in front of your house and ride with his friends," she said in an optimistic voice. Yes, in a small, square bus for special kids. My heart sank.

I was nervous as I looked at the list, second-guessing myself and wondering if this was best for him. Parents had advised me to look at all the placements the school district would give me. Placement was another new word. Was he a can of soup that had to be positioned on a shelf?

The search for a classroom started. Across a vast, empty field masquerading as a playground, a lone chair swing large enough for an adult moved slowly back and forth. The sound of the chains clinked in the background as I entered the classroom hidden in the furthest corner of the campus. Grunts came from inside the chamber; a teacher motioned me in. I expected a room with at least twenty students—there were only a handful. The few desks were scattered around the room haphazardly: one desk faced the wall, another in the center of the room, and a few were against the window. An adult, who I guessed was an aide, followed a child as he moved from one corner of the room to another.

"Time to sit and do your work," she repeated. The child moved around the classroom without pausing, ignoring the command. Close to the window was an adult who stood behind a boy slumped motionless as she manipulated his hand across a piece of paper, making marks that resembled stick figures. The teacher came towards me and introduced herself. I didn't know what to ask and blurted the first question that came to mind:

"Have you taught any students with autism?" I asked.

"Yes. Mary has autistic tendencies," she said, and looked in the direction of a girl who was jumping up and down.

I was at a loss; my mind went blank. I had no other questions.

I left the classroom hoping the next one was going to make me feel more assured that a special classroom was the best next step for Aaron.

"You worry too much," Sherman said when I described the classroom, doubting a classroom could be as dire as my description.

"I'll go with you to visit the next one. We'll find a place for him," he assured me optimistically.

A few days later we visited a classroom with a younger group—five- and six-year-olds. The children sat quietly in a semi-circle facing the teacher. She continued reading, ignoring us in the background.

"Where is the caterpillar?" she asked a young girl, and moved the book closer to her. The girl stared back at her, unresponsive, as the aide took the girl's hand and moved it towards the book.

"Yes, that's the caterpillar," the teacher said with excitement.

I had many sleepless nights during the search, filled with images of children being manipulated by those with good intentions, empty playgrounds, an adult in the bathroom scowling at a young girl as she attempted to pull up her diaper. I pushed away any thoughts of Aaron in a special school and decided to enroll him in his neighborhood kindergarten classroom.

This was 1998, when autism was not a well-known diagnosis. This lack of knowledge was evident in the school system. Special classrooms were for those with Down syndrome, cerebral palsy, and those who could not fit in a classroom for neurotypical children.

We were introducing Aaron to the external world in small doses. I wondered whether Aaron would be very different had we started intervention earlier, like the Kaufman's had with their son,

Raun, at the age of eighteen months. Now I can say probably yes, but I'll never know how he would be different. I held on to the dream that each step was bringing him closer to being a neurotypical child. I was doing the best I could and trusting each step; that's all I could manage.

Left Ear

If I touch my ear,

the left one, of course,

when I fold

the tip gently toward

my toes

I mean "No."

When I touch both tips of my

fingers,

you call them

pointer,

index,

or something else

what I want to say is

one,

or loud

or the book

waiting for me on

the kitchen chair.

You figure it out.

When I nod my head

that means "Yes."

Of course.

I wonder, when

you say

"Look at me"

is it the whiskers on your

chin,

hairs inside your nose,

the

mountain of your belly,

the veins on your right hand?

Now,

look at me.

How I touch my palms

together

namaste or

please

maybe the song I like so much

slippery fish?

Listen

to the sounds that flow

from my lips.

They are my words

like the goldfinch

outside my window

singing to those who

listen.

Asking for nothing.

Have you looked at the space

between the

bending branches

on the maple tree in your front yard?

Listened to the sound of the breeze

passing by your eager ear?

Look at the clouds

above you.

Come sit next to me.

Listen to the space between us.

Then we will talk.

Special Children

Aaron's neighborhood school was not special. I called to make an appointment to meet his teacher.

"We don't give out the names or telephone numbers of teachers," a woman at the office said, irritated by my request.

"I want to make sure she will be okay with him being there," I said in the calmest voice I could manage as I trembled with anxiety.

"She'll figure it out, I'm sure," she said.

Wasn't this a common practice? Didn't all mothers want to know where their child was?

"Can you at least give her my number?" I asked, asserting myself as much as I could without seeming rude. Growing up surrounded by boys in a male-driven culture had shut down my voice for many years. This time my son's future was at stake— I couldn't remain silent.

It became clear when other parents walked into their child's classroom for the first time on parents' night, weeks after school started. Again, I was a foreigner in a new world; this time, though, I was sharing my experience in public education with my son close to me.

Ms. Jordan's room was at the end of the corridor, overlooking the smaller of two playgrounds. I imagined Aaron coming down the slide, a smile on his face. Then suddenly a more realistic image came through: Aaron standing at the top of the play structure, observing others, involved in his own world. He was six, a bit older than most of the children in his kindergarten class, but small for his age. In some ways, he was going to fit right in.

Lyrics from a tune by the Backstreet Boys filled the halls, intermingled with chatter and laughter echoing from inside classrooms. I imagined young teachers sharing the remains of their summer adventures and wondered what the new millennium would bring. It was September 1999.

I entered Ms. Jordan's classroom; it was almost bare. A faint yellow tint bounced off the cathedral-sized walls into the center of the room where she sorted Scholastic books on a concentric table. She was a petite, wide-eyed woman, no taller than I. The wheel of the road bike she rode up the hill to school peeked from behind the curtain that separated her office space from the rest of the sprawling room. An auspicious smile greeted me with kindness and warmth. My shoulders dropped in ease. She walked around her classroom as we talked.

"Don't worry, soon these walls will be covered with paintings and life-sized drawings," she said as we both looked around the kindergarten classroom.

Nooooo, it's perfect as it is! I said to myself. Aaron would shut down when faced with too much stimulation. Didn't she realize how a child with autism would respond, or not, to all the stimulation around the room? We came from two different worlds; what was interesting and fun to neurotypical children would make Aaron retreat. I realized then how differently he experienced the world. I was there to explain Aaron's not-so-normal behavior with the hope she would understand his perceived quirkiness and be more flexible when he seemed oblivious to her requests. The barren walls were perfect as they were. Too much stimulation added one more thing for Aaron to manage.

Many years later I learned children with autism withdraw not because they are anti-social, but because they don't have the capacity to engage with unmanaged visuals or sounds. Aaron was just beginning to develop the capacity to filter out the stimulus that kept him from focusing on what was being asked of him. Sensory dysregulation can be so intense for some that it can result in extreme pain. No wonder he retreated to his own world. If given the chance and proper environment, children with autism can learn how to filter out unnecessary stimulants and self-regulate. Aaron did not have language to communicate his discomfort. I was using my voice to explain his world to others.

"I prepared this book for you," I said, and handed Ms. Jordan an illustrated story about Aaron. It was laid out in a form that six-year-olds could understand.

"I'm lucky to have a small classroom—only eighteen children!" she said with enthusiasm. My stomach tightened.

"Have you met your students?" I asked, wanting to know a bit about the children who would share her attention.

"I don't usually meet them until the first day of school," she said, with a smile that told me she was making an exception. "I think they found a good one-on-one for him," she added.

Of course, this was an exception. Aaron needed support to navigate his environment. Lydia, his one-on-one, was not a tutor, but someone who would follow him around and act like a social interpreter. But she didn't know that. Without previous training about autism or any knowledge about Aaron, how could she know how to interact with and guide an atypical child? I was hopeful that Patty would bring some guidance into this classroom and help in the understanding of his behavior.

Aaron's experience in the public education system was very different from what he was used to at home, where he had a one-student classroom with teachers totally focused on him, and where the objective was to form a personal connection with him. The public school system was new for both of us. Autism was a new world for Ms. Jordan and Lydia. In the late 1990s, autism was just beginning to be understood in mainstream culture. As the number of children with autism grew, parents demanded full inclusion in regular classrooms. This trend not only raised awareness of autism, but also brought to light the need for educators to become familiar with a growing syndrome.

Full inclusion was my dream for Aaron. In those early years, I thought being fully emerged in the day-to-day world was the next step in his development. His teacher did the best she could and met with me whenever I requested. I held on firmly to the belief that immersion was all he needed to understand his environment—not to be segregated into a special education classroom.

Memories of my own experience in a public school flooded my mind. Soon after arriving in California, my parents enrolled me in the neighborhood public school. With no understanding of the English language, I was placed in a special education classroom with children with different developmental abilities. What saved me from boredom during the long school day was the one hour I spent in a regular classroom, where fifth-grade math was taught. Immersed in the lessons about algebra, geometry, and the use of fractions, I learned English by listening to the teacher's explanations. Within six months I could understand and converse in a new language.

I held on to the belief that immersion was going to offer similar benefits; that Aaron would begin to understand his own environment, make friends, and engage in typical activities with others his age—have playdates and be invited to birthday parties. Although the school was small, and the classroom even smaller,

Aaron had a hard time adjusting to a more complex environment. He needed someone to teach him in small doses, using methods he could understand. The leap from home-schooling to a classroom was abrupt, without focused support using methods that addressed his deficits. His ability to communicate and capacity to regulate his nervous system were critical during this transitional phase. Without these, he began to retreat.

One morning, when I came to observe his classroom, he ran towards me, took my hand and led me outside. I thought he wanted to go home but instead he led me to the bathroom. Alone with him in the cool, open space, he began to cry. I wasn't sure what was going on. I knelt next to him, sensing his discomfort.

"Is something hurting?" I asked, without any response.

He stood in the middle of the large room, not wanting to move. I took his hand, and he resisted.

"I'll come back to the classroom with you," I said, trying to comfort him. He became even more determined to stay.

"Do you want to go home?" I asked. He didn't move. His behavior puzzled me. Later I realized that in the bathroom, he had found a quiet space and time to be alone. He developed a kinship for small, quiet, dim rooms and sought out places to regulate his system to be able to deal with the stimulus around him. He was seeking a safe environment. There are reasons why an environment highly charged with stimuli can be perceived by autistic individuals as threatening.

Research performed by Arian Mack and Irving Rock on intentional blindness explains that neurotypical individuals don't consciously see an object unless they are paying direct, focused attention to that object. They have an ability to filter out distractions, allowing them to focus on the immediate task. On the other hand, individuals with autism have problems filtering out sensory information and get overwhelmed when bombarded by sensory details. Aaron moved from his playroom to a classroom with screaming children, demands from the teacher, and information that was overwhelming for his system. No wonder he was shutting down.

Sensory overload delayed Aaron's typical development and added to the pressures of his overall emotional and intellectual growth. Like all children he craved physical safety, emotional communication, and the ability to navigate his social environment. Aaron struggled in what appeared to be the most supportive of environments.

What I wanted most was for him to be like others. I didn't know how to help him feel safe, communicate, or navigate his social environment. At the Options Institute, we learned how to provide a safe, holding environment supported by structure and facilitators who were present and responded to his needs. How could we bring this level of support into an educational system with expectations that don't focus on learning differences? Even the best-intentioned teacher could not fully include him in the classroom.

Neurotypical children learn by watching and mirroring the behaviors of others. Aaron was not ready to mirror others; he was doing his best to understand what was expected and asked of him. He was not ready to process language at the pace that was presented to him, and moreover, he was asked to respond to demands, questions, and social cues. He was doing the best he could in an education system that was demanding so much more.

Privileged

Intensive home-schooling continued after his day in the full-immersion classroom. We met regularly with his teacher and therapists and shared ideas on how we could smooth his immersion into the school system and make it less painful. During one of the team meetings, an important question came up: What do you want most for Aaron? We went around the table, each team member sharing their deepest desire for Aaron. These were the comments: I want him to tell me if he is in pain. I want him to be able to communicate. I want him to be able to play with others. When it came to Danielle, she responded in a way that made me pause: I want him to be happy.

What was I doing? My wishes for Aaron were a masquerade to fulfill my own needs. He didn't have a clear way to express himself; his silence had given me permission to override his feelings, as if he didn't have any of his own. Lessons from the Options Institute began to make sense. It was my own happiness I was seeking, but not through my own well-being—through Aaron's.

Aaron's education has been special in many ways. I overheard one parent say behind my back, "I wish my child had an aide." What I wanted to add was, "He'll need to take autism with that privilege." Yes, special education is just that—special. Unfortunately, equity among students who deserve truly special education is available only to a few. I was a full-time mother and advocate, fully dedicated to Aaron, with a supportive family to take care of the many needs required to raise a child with autism. I realize I, as well as Aaron, have been privileged. This thought haunted me each time I met a mother who was struggling and not able to provide for the basic needs of her child. My heart ached over stories of a mother who had taken her life and that of her child when she could not cope anymore. Over the years, parents have created organizations to support each other on the complex journey of parenthood.

The year at the public school was difficult for me; I can only imagine how arduous it must have been for Aaron. From a distance, everything looked wonderful. I made several friendships in the community and, for the first time Aaron was able to participate in activities that were easily accessible to neurotypical children. He was invited to birthday parties, picnics, and a performance by the San Francisco Symphony. Because of his specialness, I was able to arrange box seats at Symphony Hall for a performance of *Peter and the Wolf*. His kindergarten class shared in the benefit.

His school year was carefully managed. Ms. Jordan prepared lesson plans for her special student, different from the ones she prepared for the rest of the class. She made time to meet regularly with me and his home-school teachers. But it was not enough. The environment was not set up for individual teaching—time given to one student would take away from the rest of the children in the class. As small as the classroom was, it was set up to teach those who could benefit from a group experience.

Our society would be transformed if each child received an education tailored to their needs. How different would our school system be if every child was met where they were—where every student was treated as special? Imagine a world where the educational system focused on each child's physical, social, and emotional development.

It's taken years for Aaron to feel safe in public and around neurotypical peers and to express himself in his own unique way.

At the end of his kindergarten year, it was clear full inclusion was not going to work for Aaron. Tears flowed when he said goodbye to Ms. Jordan and Lydia, his one-on-one classroom assistant. We passed the vast playground where his PE teacher had made modifications so he, too, could play soccer with the other boys. Daisy, a young girl who had been his friend since the first day of school, handed Aaron a book called *My Friend Aaron*, which he treasures to this day. The children in the classroom did the best they knew how to include him in every activity. Over the past twenty years and numerous studies around socialization, it has become clear that simply being near neurotypical peers is not likely to produce favorable outcomes for children with autism. Thoughtful planning is needed to teach peers how to get the attention of and engage someone like Aaron. Integrated playgroups were not recognized in mainstream educational settings. Ready or not, we were determined to continue the journey in the public-school environment and find a place where Aaron belonged.

Although the year in public school was challenging, I was left with the hope that people have a genuine intention to do what's right. Teachers need support from the school system and parents. Unfortunately, unspoken fiscal budgets guide the decisions that impact children in the public school system.

I kept going back to my first years as a young girl in a foreign country, striving to gain a sense of belonging. It was a slow process through some very lonely years in my teens. I could only imagine the sense of isolation Aaron was experiencing as he reached the critical age of seven, when the world was supposed to start making sense and social interactions were an important part of understanding his world. Aaron's sense of belonging was compromised, and I felt powerless. In addition to growing up as an only child at home, Aaron was also a unique child in his community. How could he ever develop his own sense of belonging? I feared for his soul.

"Soul has to do with the way a human being belongs to their world, their work, or their human community. Where there is little sense of belonging there is little sense of soul. The soulful qualities of life depend on these qualities of belonging. It seems to me that human beings are always desperate to belong to something larger than themselves.

"When they do not feel this belonging they not only feel as if they are running in place, they quite often feel as if they are dying in place. Without belonging no attempt to coerce enthusiasm or imagination from us can be sustained for long."

—*The Heart Aroused,* David Whyte

Out of Sync

The park was an extension of our backyard, just blocks away from our home. Maybe there Aaron could learn how to be like other children. It was a green oasis brimming with activity, where I would encourage him to play with toddlers who were regulars at the playground. We passed a young girl pushing her little sister on the swing, then came up to a young boy giggling while sliding down a slide. In the distance, the familiar voice of the train conductor could be heard: All aboard! Aaron was the last child to settle into a bucket-sized seat before the train started its short journey around the track.

San Mateo's Central Park was alive with the smell of popcorn from the snack bar and children shouting joyfully as they ran around the flagpole in the middle of the grass-covered field. A visit to the park was part of the daily routine with Abuela. After breakfast, she prepared a snack, buckled Aaron in the stroller and headed out for a morning stroll. This day I joined my mother and Aaron on their daily stroll to the park. We sat on the bench engulfed by laughter coming from the playground and kept an eye on Aaron as he played alone in the sandbox.

"Do you think he likes other children?" Mother asked. Her brow furrowed as we watched him dribble sand from one hand into the sandbox.

"I think so," I said, somewhat unsure of my answer.

From afar he looked like a typical child playing in the sand. His hands, like small buckets, dipped into the sandy pool; palms down, he watched intently as the granules fell through his fingers.

He was absorbed in the miracle in front of him, repeating the movement over and over. I called his name, wanting to break the hypnotic trance. There was no response. Suddenly he got up and ran towards an empty metal swing that was still moving. I followed him, curious about what drew his attention. I froze when I saw him run towards the swing, thinking he would stop when he saw it coming towards him. He didn't stop but allowed the swing to hit the side of his head and knock him to the sand. For years I've carried the guilt of not protecting him from the impact of the metal swing.

Months after we began intervention, when Aaron was around four, I began to become familiar with the habitual behaviors of children with autism, and realized that what could be mistaken as play was something else. I began to observe him through a different lens. He was experiencing the world from a different lens than neuro-typical children. How was autism impacting the way he experienced the world? Was it the movement of the sand, the warmth, or how the light reflected against each granule that kept his attention? What was it about the swing that drew him towards it? The movement? The clinking sound of the chains? Or was he late in responding to the child who had left the swing?

A note in the white binder led me to a book that opened my mind about Aaron's behavior. *The Out-of-Sync Child*, by Carol Stock Kranowitz, describes sensory dysregulation. Her explanation and examples of a disorganized sensory system gave me insight as to what was causing the inconsistent behavior I was observing. When overstimulated by the sounds or visuals around him, Aaron withdrew to a corner. Other times he sought extra stimulation, like the impromptu rush towards the swing.

His kindergarten teacher and peers were also perplexed by his behavior. While rehearsing in the auditorium for a performance of The Gingerbread Man, Aaron hid behind the curtain and refused to join his friends.

"I thought he liked music," Daisy said. She had formed a connection with Aaron since the beginning of the school year, and they had formed a sweet friendship. Aaron seemed to enjoy her company. Why didn't he want to join in and dance like he did in the classroom? From the stage, the voices reverberated through a large, open hall and the view towards the empty seats in the dark auditorium may have felt uncomfortable.

"Why is he by himself in the corner?" Daisy asked as she walked towards Aaron. She took his hand and led him to the center of the stage. "You can be the cow in the pasture," she said. He followed, with some hesitancy. While I observed Aaron's behavior from afar, I was making space for my own ambivalence to show up: Did I want him to be self-directed and take his own initiative, or was there some comfort in leading him around so he could look normal? Were my hopes for him in conflict with his own? I wanted to see him like other children—was that what he wanted? Was I imposing my own wishes on him? I continued working with these questions that were the source of much of my own inner work.

What he needed at that time in his life was an occupational therapist who understood his sensory regulation needs. I, too, was learning the roles and benefits of different interventions and began to understand that the function of occupational therapy was not to teach him how to hold a pencil, as one therapist told me, but to help him regulate his sensory system so he could function in his daily life. His senses were disorganized; this was hindering his ability to play, to socialize, and to learn from interactions with other children. I began to understand what was meant by "Play is children's work." Aaron's disorganized sensory system made his most basic daily functions extremely difficult.

Kranowitz explains sensory problems as the inability to modulate one's sensory system. Even Aaron's most basic movements, like walking, were compromised. At times he craved sensory input by seeking movement, and he'd suddenly run without warning. I began to understand. These responses no longer seemed random; instead, they pointed to the way Aaron experienced his world.

When left alone, I'd find him next to a window where the sun streamed in, watching the rays of light coming between his fingers as he strummed them on his cheek. Music was both soothing and stimulating, sometimes lulling him to sleep and other times exciting him to the point of being overwhelmed. As he got older and his sensory system was better regulated, he'd know when to turn the music off or say, "No" when Sherman began to play the piano. It was a great relief when Aaron became able to ask for what he needed.

It wasn't just the need for stimulation that was keeping him from participating in daily life; autism compromised his mental capacity to plan and focus attention, to remember simple instructions, and to juggle multiple tasks. Low muscle tone led to a high tolerance for pain and temperature. Aaron's internal world was scrambled. No wonder his attention was inward and social cues didn't enter his awareness. Unable to filter unnecessary details, his social environment became confusing.

What was most distressing for me was that he seldom cried, complained, or asked for comfort by being held. He used repetitive behavior to regulate himself and withdraw from what was too much to handle. Self-stimulation provided some form of comfort and information to his body.

Over the years, I've seen up-close the many strategies autistic children use to self-regulate. Some of them are bizarre and even dangerous. Some children have limited food preferences, like the boy who would eat only French fries, while others have extreme attraction to certain sounds, scents, and sensory stimulation. What I find distressing is knowing that many non-verbal individuals are unable to express discomfort, so their internal, unobservable sensations go unaddressed. What seems like idiosyncratic behavior to the untrained eye may be a way to regulate and create order within their system and connect with their inner world. As I was slowly drawn into Aaron's world, my pain became unbearable.

I began to understand how I was coping with my own pain.

Knowing the Unknown

It was an atypically clear summer morning on the coast when a phone call from an unrecognized caller caused me to pull to the side of the road within sight of a sprawling pumpkin patch. Roxanne was the life coach whom I'd met in a workshop a few months before. She had an opening in her schedule the following Tuesday morning. I paused before I said yes to coaching, a new experience. I was familiar with therapy, being around treatment methods that supported Aaron's growth. I understood therapy to be a fix for an unwanted condition—autism. I was willing to give this new form of therapy a try to see if it could bring more ease into my life.

Roxanne's office was conveniently located a few blocks away from Wings, a school for children with autism I had started in 2001 with a group of educators. Aaron was eight years old then, and I finally felt he was supported by people who understood him and were in line with his needs. The school was small, with one other autistic boy in the classroom. The teachers had experience in autism and were totally focused on what the two students needed to thrive.

I, on the other hand, was overwhelmed with the demands of starting and managing a new venture: a school that, although meant for Aaron, was going to serve many other students like him. What was I thinking?

Morning glory vines in full bloom against a fence led me from a narrow pathway to Roxanne's front door. I turned the completed intake form around and around in my hand until it resembled a paper telescope. I had answered all the questions as best I could except for one: What would you do if you knew you could not fail?

A woman with fair skin and kind, blue eyes greeted me with a smile. I then felt as at ease as I had the first time I'd met her.

Taped to the front of her office door was a sign: EXPECT SOMETHING WONDERFUL TO HAPPEN. I wondered what that would be.

I could see through the window to the outside, where sailboats were moving away from the harbor. After we sat on the large winged chairs, she lit a candle and looked up at me. The silence between us allowed me to take a breath and settle into the room.

"What brings you here?" she asked. I paused and searched for an answer.

"Well, I don't know why I get anxious when I'm about to meet someone for the first time," I said. I was surprised by my response. She jotted something on a yellow paper pad. Silence filled the room, and I felt the need to say something.

"Well, not really; what I'm feeling is lonely, deep down inside," I said, holding back tears. The words that came out, again, surprised me. I had never expressed these emotions to a total stranger.

"Go on," she said.

"Each time I hear a doctor say I don't know, my stomach tightens."

She looked at me for a moment, waiting for me to continue.

"I guess what really brings me here is…I'm scared I won't be able to take care of my son." I could barely hear myself finish the sentence. "One night I woke up with chest pains and thought I was having a heart attack." I recalled the night when I ended up in the emergency room.

"Anything else?" she asked in a slow, kind voice.

The expression of a long-held fear gave me some relief. A foghorn in the background sounded, and soon our session was over. The following week I returned and began our session by recapping my relationship with my mother.

"Tell me more," she said when I paused.

"I'm in conflict all the time. I need her help and yet it drives me crazy when she shows up unannounced at all hours of the day."

The soft sound of the foghorn in the background calmed me down. Memories of my childhood in El Salvador flooded in. Why wasn't I bothered by unexpected visitors to our home back then? I was never surprised to find a bowl of mangos on the dining table, wondering who had stopped by on the way back from the market. It all changed when we came to California. I began to feel separate, different from others—there were those who belonged in this country and then there was me, trying to make sense of how to be one of them. I was a visitor in a country that was not my own.

"Tell me more about the heart attack," she asked.

I began to recollect that night, giving her details of how I was suddenly awakened by chest pain, the ride in the ambulance, the emergency room...

She gently interrupted me. "So, what are you afraid of?" she asked. I sat in silence as the foghorn sounded.

"I'm afraid that..." I said, and broke down sobbing. Tears didn't often come easily, but that morning, the questions penetrated the core of my fear. There was an unknown I had tapped into—my own unknowing. The wake-up call was loud and clear. Something had to change. I was responding to a fear I needed to face. Again.

On that day, I began a journey of self-discovery, unraveling layers and layers of beliefs, beginning a new relationship to my unconscious and conscious self. I realized that, after forty-seven years on this earth, I knew little about myself. I was introduced to the Enneagram, a map for getting to know myself by observing my own behavior.

Years of careful evaluation of Aaron's behavior had given me some insight into why he did certain things. What if I used the same mental process to evaluate my own behavior? I began to learn, slowly—very slowly—how to disidentify myself from my behavior and see it as the response of my psychological structure. If I understood what that structure was, maybe I could understand myself.

What I learned over the following years was to dance between introspection and observation: looking inward at my sensations, emotions, and thoughts, and looking outward at my behavior. It was through this constant inner and outer awareness that I began to gain insight into my own beliefs, behaviors, and motivations. My relationship to myself and to life began anew.

Three Marriages

The air smelled of dry seaweed. I rolled down the car window and breathed it in. Far off, I could make out the wet-suited surfers as they patiently waited for the next wave. Aaron's thick head of black hair was visible through the rearview mirror—we looked towards the open ocean. Another school year was about to begin. This time, I was responsible for guiding the curriculum and choosing his teachers.

"It's not going to be easy," Sherman said when I told him I was ready to start a school.

"It's hard enough to deal with the teachers who don't even know what autism is," I said, determined to move ahead with the plan.

Each September my stomach tightened with anxiety as I faced another milestone. Was there any progress? I would make sure he made progress in his struggles to communicate and be more a part of his world.

"Are you sure you want to do this?" the woman on the other end of the phone asked.

"We're going to give this school a chance," I said.

"What? I'm not sure I got that," she said as I noticed my voice becoming quieter with each word. The fear of failing my son was nagging at me. The school intended to help Aaron and others like him.

"We're going to try to make it work," I repeated, raising my voice, confident that the administrator heard me.

For what seemed like hours, time stopped as I listened to my inner voice. I realized the woman on the other end was giving me time to change my mind.

"You realize you're giving up your rights," she warned. I was giving up Aaron's rights to be part of the public education system. Deep inside, I knew we could do better.

We opened the school in 2001, after planning and visualizing what an ideal classroom and school would look like for Aaron and others like him. A group of educators from San Francisco State University met to plan and create a school that would place the child at the center of every decision. We felt the need to find radical ways of engaging children with autism and knew it must be a two-way learning process. The child would guide the educators to a deeper understanding of his needs; the educator, in turn, would reflect and respond with the appropriate teaching method for the child. It looked like a typical classroom, led by a special education teacher and supported by a progressive speech-language pathologist. Their focus: to inspire in Aaron the desire to communicate. Eventually, other children would become part of the school community.

Years later, I learned to consciously step inside myself and listen to my inner voice. It would guide me towards the next step. I became able to get in touch with that voice and recognize when I was facing a step I didn't want to take. Opening the school was something I wasn't prepared to do, but a step I needed to take. Before I learned to listen to that voice, angst and fear propelled me into action. Action in any form dulled my angst—at least for a short while.

I had no idea what I was doing. As I led the effort to set up a new school, I slowly stepped into a new vocation: school administrator of Aaron's education. It was a mission larger than me or Aaron, one that would impact the lives of other children. It was like flying solo for the first time, with my family in the plane. Ignorance blinded me to future roadblocks. I had fallen in love with the possibilities that lay ahead.

We could see the entrance to the Wilkinson School from Highway 1 as we passed it on the way to Princeton Harbor to pick up fresh crab off the boats, never noticing the small Cape Cod blue building. That September morning was different; everything around me had an accentuated aliveness.

To anyone looking at the school we called Wings, two full-time teachers in a one-room schoolhouse with one student may have appeared excessive. It soon became a prototype for a classroom that would soon be open to many. Inside was a single desk and a semi-circular table surrounded by five small chairs, where group activities took place with children from the neighboring school.

The Wilkinson School, adjacent to Wings, was a small private school for neurotypical students. Children from the school visited Aaron's classroom and joined him during circle time, Aaron's favorite part of the six-hour school day. His smile and wide-eyed delight were clear signs of joy. I was unsure whether it was the music and songs or the other children that gave him such pleasure. I hoped he would become engaged with both.

The Wilkinson campus was a non-traditional private school, from kindergarten to eighth grade, all encompassed in one large building sectioned into six classrooms. Two teachers shared a full academic curriculum plus drama, music, and art. The Wings classroom was within steps of the Wilkinson campus, where Aaron shared the playground and picnic tables that overlooked a wide, sandy beach.

Like the pelicans that hovered overhead, Aaron was about to take a deep dive into a new way of learning and being with others. The teachers were also on their personal journeys. They created an individual curriculum for each child who came to Wings. Then they facilitated a social environment where they could all learn together as a group. It was a deep dive into education, self-reflection, and observation of their students' behaviors.

Aaron's education suddenly took a different course. Students became the source for the teaching methods. Functional skills: washing hands, saying hello to others, and commenting on the environment were the basis of each task. Behavior gave us clues and led to understanding deeper motivators, both for the teachers and the students.

Wings began to attract educators who were receptive to the different ways children with autism learned, and who led the students, step by step, towards inner growth. The student was both the giver and receiver of information, and the educators were observers of their own behavior as well as that of their students. There were no problems to fix—only the next question to ask.

What changed my view of education was a conversation I had with a young intern in the San Francisco State School of Special Education who was also a new immigrant from Singapore.

"I see Aaron's struggles as the same as mine," she said in broken English, when I asked her why she wanted to be Aaron's tutor. "I know what I want to say, but the words don't always come easy," she continued.

Within days, she and Aaron formed a close bond. Aaron paid focused attention to her instructions, and he was happy to see her. That personal connection was an essential key to learning. That bond created trust and a safe place for Aaron to learn and thrive. That young intern later became an exceptional special education teacher.

On that September morning in 2001, I started a journey into the complex field of education. Many inequalities in how we educate our youth became evident as I interacted with school officials. My motivation was to give Aaron the best chance to be who he was and be seen as a unique individual. Until then, the teaching methods I had learned focused on working towards being normal. That was no longer important to me.

The word "placement" has always bothered me. Yet, it was an essential word in IDEA, the law that allowed opportunities for individuals with disabilities to learn next to their neurotypical peers. "Placement" accentuated the belief that people with disabilities didn't have the capacity to make their own decisions, a partial truth. All individuals can learn to make decisions to the best of their ability. I noticed that some educators, unconsciously, view students with different abilities as passive participants in their future. During the years that followed as a self-taught educator, I met teachers who could see beyond the limitations and nurture the abilities of their students. I firmly believe that until we dissociate the word "special" from education, children will continue to be underserved by our efforts to educate.

Having been involved in education for over twenty years now, I'm grateful for this new relationship with what it means to be a teacher.

In his book The Three Marriages, David Whyte suggests we ask these two questions before entering a love or work relationship:

Is the one I'm pursuing my true love?

Is my work real and is it any help to others?

Without knowing it, the education field became my newfound profession. I was about to begin a courtship with my son, my work, and myself.

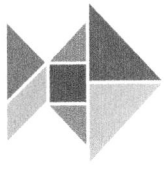

PART 3
A Way Through

"Our plans never turn out as tasty as reality."

—Ram Dass

Atonal Symphony

And then came summer.

Wings, a new school, and unfamiliar schoolmates: the twin girls from Dublin, whose parents moved to California to find a sense of hope—anything to reach their severely autistic daughters. A boy from Kobe, whose family was transferred to San Francisco. Another student, who in a public school had spent the six-hour day under a table in an empty gym.

"You gotta take this kid," the legal advocate who visited the classroom said. "The school doesn't know what to do with him."

"He has no place to go, and his mom is losing it." She pleaded with me to give the boy a chance. A week into the summer session, the boy's mother went to Wings and observed her son from a distance. She peeked from behind a shed in the outside play area. As she looked over at her son, exchanging glances with another boy as they threw a ball back and forth, her face began to glow and tears poured down her face. Could others understand how a small act of normal behavior would lighten a heart? It softened mine, and I knew I had found my calling.

I began to feel a profound responsibility for the children and their parents, something I had not expected. The small schoolhouse was barely big enough for eight students and as many staff. Saying no became a practice that called on being true to myself and to the parents who were certain the school was where their child needed to be.

Families were happy to see their children in a place that cared for them. There was a one-to-one staff-to-student ratio, which gave me a sense there was enough capacity to take care of each child's individual needs.

Three young interns were there to learn from more senior staff—a special ed teacher, a speech pathologist, and an occupational therapist. We were all taking part in an experiment where the teachers were conductors of an atonal symphony, showing the students various instruments to choose from and make their own unique music. They were teaching in a new modality, where the children were engaged, and helping them build a sense of self and have fun.

What appeared to be a small class of eight students was an intensely active and demanding environment: children ages seven to ten who were all in need of intensive support to engage in activities that, to neurotypical children, were seen as natural, like going to the bathroom and washing their hands. Teachers seemed to "get" their students. They focused on getting to know the child and letting go of preconceived ideas about autism. Trust was the basis of their interactions. Once they connected, the child would follow when asked and lead when there was space for that to happen naturally.

Aaron, one of eight students, didn't mind sharing the teachers' attention with other students. He was learning in his own way and enjoying being in a lively environment.

The boy who had been under the table in the gym at his previous school, soon became accustomed to the freedom of his new environment and developed a habit of bolting and running away towards the street. Teachers gathered after each school day to brainstorm new ways to teach self-regulation, communication, and especially, how to engage with the students and meet them where they were. The questions were not simple: How do you encourage spontaneous communication? How do you teach children to take initiative? What makes us want to act and what gives us the will to stop? Is it biological, learned, or both? How does autism impact these questions?

The students brought their temperament, communication style, sensory needs, coping strategies, and passionate likes and dislikes. A boy from India was the most verbal—unlike most of his classmates, he would not stop talking. What on the surface sounded like coherent language was a stream of nonsensical words. It took a patient and insightful teacher to listen and be sensitive to his needs. The boy felt heard and that made all the difference. The twin girls were non-verbal, shy, and reserved. Each chose to go to a different corner of the room, one twirling her hair into knots and the other looking intently out the window. A young woman teacher looked out the window and shared the view; a connection began to form.

Repetition reinforced practical skills, which became tricky because repetition could easily turn into a stim, at least for Aaron. He quickly learned to type music on his communication device we called a Talker. At first, he was praised and rewarded with music. It then became a repetitive request that kept him from being engaged in other activities, so the next step was to teach him that communication was a two-way interaction. Asking for his favorite activity turned into an interactive exchange:

"Music, please," Aaron said on his Talker.

"Which song do you want to hear?" his teacher asked.

"Music," he said again.

"Do you want to listen to 'Listen to the Water' or 'Row, Row, Row Your Boat'?" the teacher asked.

"Water," he responded.

"Okay!" the teacher said as she turned on the song "Listen to the Water" on the music box.

Circles of communication expanded with every request.

The children didn't mind the cramped and boisterous classroom, except for Aaron, whose favorite activity was Quiet Time. When given a choice of activity, he'd take his books and plop himself down on a chair in the make-shift library. While others played on the playground or jumped up and down until it was time to go home, the boy from Kobe was quiet, except when he was playing with his building blocks. Verbal utterances followed each placement of a wooden block.

It took weeks for the children to be ready to go on beach walks as a group. They were learning to regulate themselves, follow the teacher, and stay close to the group. The teachers were learning the idiosyncrasies of each student and planning for the unexpected. Smiles began to glow on faces when the icon with an image of the ocean was placed on the schedule. It was time for a walk to the beach. The boy who once spent most of the time under the table now happily shared space with his classmates, repeating the activities of the day.

"Today we're going to the beach, to the beach, to the beach, today we're going to the beach," he said.

No one seemed to mind his repetitive speech except Aaron, who would cover his ears as the boy's voice escalated in pitch and volume. I was encouraged by Aaron's tolerance; not long ago, he was the only one in the classroom. Now, he was sharing a small space with classmates and teachers.

The energy from the school day continued to fill the classroom after the children went home. Staff meetings went on for hours, consumed by thorough debriefings of each student's day.

Discussions revolved around each child's behavior, communicative intent, preferred activities, and academic progress, giving the teachers a critical insight into the students' motivations. Also, teachers became students as they learned the complexities of managing a school. Some teachers openly shared their challenges and talked about the impact the classroom was having on their well-being. It was working us all, personally and emotionally. I took part in the meetings as the teachers reviewed, discussed, and argued the different ways of teaching and treating a range of behaviors, problems, and questions, with acute care. Conflicting views were placed on the table and discussed openly. How to deal with a specific behavior was always part of a conversation that led to the next steps in teaching a new skill.

"Houston, we have a problem," was a recurring message often left on my answering machine.

"Don't touch that!" Sherman said one evening as we were ready to sit down for dinner. We agreed that I would not answer phone calls after we sat down for dinner. Even though I agreed, my mind kept going in circles into the evening.

The complexity of autism was clearly evident in the few children who passed through the doors in those early years. One child's strength was another's deficit. Teaching was about observing, listening, and responding to their needs as they came up. It was a process that required a quiet space inside ourselves so we could hear the silence between the words.

Summer went by quickly. The teachers were exhausted, and yet the children were not ready for summer school to end. That summer, it became certain that Wings was going to grow. These children needed a safe space where they could be themselves. The following school year, 2002, we searched for a larger and more accessible location in the Bay Area.

Guernica

We stepped onto the dirt path that protected pedestrians from traffic on both sides of the park. The *Paseo del Prado*, two thoroughfares with the same name, sandwiched the park from the east and west sides. We were groggy from the polar flight from San Francisco to Madrid. Only one place could keep my eyes open until the evening, when my head would plunge eagerly into a pillow and sleep would synchronize my circadian rhythm—we were feet away from the Prado Museum when I saw the sign: *CERRADO*.

I had planned to give my time to one painting inside the shrine of Spanish masters: *Las Meninas* by Velazquez. Each time I looked at this work, I would get lost in the different viewpoints: was I, the observer, looking into the painting, or were the *meninas* looking at me? Who was observing and who was being observed? The work remains an enigma. Understanding the artist's intention and my own discovery of the symbolism continues to work my curiosity. The museum was not just closed for the day but for months ahead as it endured a massive restoration.

What had started as a crisp, clear day turned into a disappointment that May morning. We decided to take a stroll behind the museum and follow the gravel pathway dotted by emerging crocus to the *Parque del Buen Retiro*.

I remember feeling empty, tired, and full of angst. I was looking forward to being engulfed by the masterpieces in the museum and, for a moment, forget that Aaron was thousands of miles away. If there was an emergency, I couldn't jump in and fix it. After a few moments of anxious breathing, I was able to calm down and wake up to the reality and luxury of time, undisturbed by dead-lines or meetings and without a destination in mind.

Sherman and I walked together in silence under a canopy of maple trees not knowing what to say to each other, like two people on a first date. We hadn't been alone, away from Aaron, for eight years. This was the second time we'd left him. Voices coming from a group of children in the middle of a green open area gave me a sudden energy spike. I thought of Aaron, back home in his new school, and wondered if he was playing with the kids or standing in a corner, away from the crowd.

We passed a group of hefty, grandmotherly women on cement benches, gossiping with the most serious frowns.

"I wonder if they're still awake," I said to Sherman.

"Don't worry, he's fine," he answered as he unfolded a map.

"I was just thinking we should let them know we made it here," I said.

"We can call them in a few days. Don't bother them," Sherman said as he studied the map.

Traces of cigarette smoke led the way to a popular spot in the park, the *Palacio de Cristal*. Pods of people sat around the plaza; others sauntered around the fountain. The beauty of the building again awakened me. What a grand substitute for a visit to the Prado. We walked, undisturbed, into the museum. There was another surprise inside: *Guernica*, Picasso's sprawling masterpiece, was temporarily on exhibit.

I wasn't expecting to see this monumental and disturbing painting. A handful of serious viewers walked around the salon, some with hands behind their backs, some covering their faces as they took in the monochromatic depiction of the 1937 bombing of the small Basque town. Emotions swelled up in me as I looked over the images of the victims on the canvas. Sharp tongues and rays of light coming from a light bulb illuminating a distressed horse hit me like exploding grenades. I walked back and forth, covering the length of the twenty-foot painting time and time again, leaving each jolt of pain on the canvas and moving to the next.

A detail on the far edge of the canvas stopped me. The image of Michelangelo's *Pieta* came to mind, the work that brings tears to anyone who can bear to sit with the tender pain embedded in the flowing marble: Mary, holding her son on her lap, shares an intimate moment in which love and surrender meet. Picasso's images are violent. They allow for a sharp, piercing pain to enter our hearts. In a detail, a mother sits with her dying child. A single, naked breast points down towards the baby on her lap. Her face looks upward in grief, her mouth opened by a sharp, triangular tongue that points up to the heavens in anger.

It took years to process the pain I felt for myself and for my son. It started as grief over a normal, imagined childhood stolen away from us. It took years to allow that the illusion of normalcy was just that: an illusion. Yet the pain was real, and the falling grenades pierced open my heart so I could experience the love of the child that was given to me.

Polarities

It was an unexpected experience of both spaciousness and peace, and feeling the pain that arises from our human frailties. In some ways, it was a typical morning when I made breakfast, packed lunch for Aaron, and headed out to school. He was buckled in his seat at 8:00 a.m., ready for the second week of a new school year at Wings.

I stopped at the Shell station before turning onto Highway 92, which led over the hill to the coastal town of El Granada. As I pulled up to the pump, I noticed a woman standing in front of her car, hand covering her mouth, eyes wide with fear, unmoving as she listened to the news report coming from the car radio. I knew she had just heard the news that shook the world that morning. The Twin Towers had toppled, and another plane had just hit the Pentagon.

I hugged Aaron tightly that morning when I said goodbye. My eyes lingered on him as he walked towards the stack of books waiting for him on the only desk in the classroom. He was safe there. Teacher Amy and I exchanged looks. Did Aaron sense the emotions that engulfed him on that unforgettable morning, beyond anyone's comprehension? How could I ever fully explain what had happened on the other side of our country?

On edge, I felt the need to be comforted by nature and drove a few miles north to the Fitzgerald Marine Reserve. As I arrived, I was entering a refuge from the unexplainable events. The morning was brisk, the sky blue—a perfect September day on the West Coast. Seagulls hovered over me as I stepped down a path leading to a sheltered beach. Images of the rubble, smoke, and fire replayed over and over in my head as I dipped my feet into a wading pool, careful not to step on the spiny sea urchins covered by gentle waves of the cool ocean water. Moisture from the morning fog was beginning to evaporate from the rocks, and driftwood was scattered on the beach where I began my walk. Images of men in business suits running away from the debris and ash besieged me.

The sound of the foam touching the sand calmed me for an instant, until the violent encounter of the waves against boulders brought me back. It was possible to hold the beauty around me and the dread that was on the surface all around us. A gentle breeze woke me up to the smell of seaweed. I was alive. Years later, I learned it was possible to hold several conflicting emotions at what appeared to be a simultaneous time—coming into awareness of my body's sensations was the opening that allowed me to accept both anguish and solace—guilt slowly receded into the background.

Motherhood had been a blur. I wondered how my life would have been different had Aaron been a neurotypical child; he would be in third or fourth grade, listening to a counselor as she attempted to explain what had happened that morning in Manhattan. I had lost touch with normal; on that September day, I felt in community with others. The previous five years had been consumed with constant plans for the classroom and teachers who could understand an autistic child and then prepare lesson plans. We had tried oral therapy—a manipulation of Aaron's tongue and palette that might have helped him articulate and eventually communicate. Aaron had joined social groups where neurotypical children were his guides during play interaction. All along, I had been hopeful that soon he would have friends—real friends who appreciated the person he was and would play with him as they would with other children. I had questioned if he would ever have friends. Teachers had taught him how to read, so he could type words on his typing machines and communicate with others. Mine was a selfish wish:

to hear his voice so he could tell me his dreams and what toys he wanted for Christmas and what silly costume he wanted to wear for Halloween. What did he think about the insanity that led planes into the skyscrapers that morning?

Friends asked, "How is he doing?" Underneath the question was a curiosity: Was Aaron becoming more like other children— talking, reading, or playing baseball; was he becoming normal?

As I walked down the beach, I passed a young mother with a dazed look on her face as she sat on a log, watching her toddler chase his dog into the waves. The toddler laughed as a shower of saltwater from his furry friend's back bathed him. The pain and joy of the scene encouraged me to continue until I came to a wall of boulders that blocked my path. Should I scale them or return to my car? Other than getting Aaron from school that afternoon, I had nothing else planned, so I attempted the climb to discover what was on the other side.

The smell of fresh kelp seeped through cracks in the rocks; mini crabs ran from one crevice to the next, dodging the water coming in from high tide. Then I felt the force of the waves against the rocks and I moved slowly, carefully placing my feet on each boulder.

Morning soon turned to afternoon, and I felt my face burn from exposure to the sun. A small beach house with an open window gave me another glimpse of the normal world: an older man stood motionless, staring at a television screen. I walked back to the car and headed towards the school where Aaron was waiting for me. For him, it was just another day at school. Aaron was safe in the schoolhouse, far from the chaos. That morning I felt part of a larger world—one where we all shared the pain of our human existence.

Meteor

Aaron waited patiently at the door of the schoolhouse for Abuelo to pick him up as he did daily while Abuela prepared lunch for him, which she neatly placed on the table, ready for him when he entered through the kitchen door: cherry tomatoes in a small rice bowl and grilled chicken with ketchup next to white rice.

This afternoon, Aaron's schedule had changed. He was part of a discussion about his new communication device called a Lightwriter. It was a simple keyboard with an elongated screen above the keys, where each letter appeared as it was typed. When the return key was pressed, a robotic voice, sounding very much like Stephen Hawking's machine, enunciated the words.

While Aaron played on the iMac in the corner of the classroom, Alison, an optimistic speech pathologist, waited for the rest of us to join her, where the small machine took its kingly place at the center of a conference table. She eagerly led us through the multistep strategy. Her plan was designed to teach Aaron how to use this new device. The Lightwriter was going to give Aaron a "voice." She was certain of that.

Aaron continued playing, uninterrupted, as his teacher and I got ready to learn.

"Let's start with introducing him to words he already knows," she said with a smile. Music, song, dance, juice, park, and beach were at the top of the list. "I'll guide him through the keyboard using hand-over-hand. It's important he gets used to this device, so it needs to be next to him at all times," she said in a more serious voice, wanting us all to take responsibility for this new role.

A thick strap was meant to go securely around his shoulder.

Alison read out the first lesson plan: she was going to teach him to spell, first on the computer, and then transfer the skill to the Lightwriter.

We spent the next half hour talking about some basic rules: what to call the machine, how we were going to refer to it when we talked to Aaron, and how to make sure other kids also took it seriously.

"They need to understand this is his voice and not a toy," she said, as her brows furrowed slightly. It was important to use the proper language.

Where is your voice?

Get your Talker.

Use your words.

After some strategizing, Alison was ready to introduce Aaron to the new device.

"Aaron, come join us and see your Talker," Alison said in a high-pitched voice. Aaron didn't move; instead, he continued playing a Sesame Street game on the computer. Janice, his teacher, went over and enticed him to take a break and join us at the big table, where we were discussing his "voice."

The Talker was placed in front of Aaron.

"What do you think?" Alison asked, moving the Talker closer.

Aaron reached for the machine and quickly typed, "Done." He then walked back to the computer and continued the game that was interrupted by his teacher.

We looked at each other, our mouths half-open. Alison took her notes, crumpled them up in a small paper ball, and threw them in the garbage.

I realized at that moment that Aaron was like a meteor coming towards us. He had his own path. We were not only trying to predict the trajectory of his future, but also trying to guide its course. The force heading towards me was constantly changing, and I needed to change with him. It was clear he had much to teach us. Our job was to become quiet, listen, and watch. He was moving fast. Sometimes he disappeared behind a cloudy sky, but he was always there. I needed to be present, vigilant, and ready to act when he landed.

Blue Mockingbird

Oh, Mama, welcome back

let me hear your voice.

Fly with me.

If I could, I would

tell you

when my words arrived

tonight

scattered in the fields

turning to dust

into soil

so you can follow

the light of

the new moon.

Someday

a clay flute

will whisper

what the mockingbird knows.

Aware of Being Aware

Who would have thought that four grown men bobbing their heads from side to side to the beat of the music like a single metronome would keep hundreds of three-year-olds engaged? They wore identical mock-turtleneck shirts, each a different primary color. It was 2003 when The Wiggles performed at Foothill College in Silicon Valley in one of their first U.S. tours. Every seat in the auditorium appeared to be taken by toddlers wiggling their tiny behinds with anxious anticipation. We took our assigned seats, from which we had a full view of the stark stage.

I stepped over bitty legs stretched out like branches; Aaron's hand coupled tightly with mine. I could barely hear my own voice in the midst of the thunderous screeches of children's voices. I'm not sure if Aaron heard what I was saying.

"Right here, Aaron," Nina said as she grabbed the edge of his shirt and led him down to the chair meant for him. It had been Nina's idea to see The Wiggles and she had asked her mom if Aaron could come along. At four, she already had a keen sense of what she wanted.

Lights buzzed around us. Clusters of fanatical children settled into oversized velvet chairs as the room began to darken.

"Shushhhh!" echoed all around us.

"Can you stay quiet just for a second?" a young mother in the row behind us asked exasperatedly.

"It will be a while till I can say that to Aaron," I mumbled.

Miriam rubbed my shoulder softly as she gazed at Aaron, slumped in the chair next to me.

"The Wiggles will be here any minute! Sit up so you can see them!" Nina said with excitement.

Although they were six years apart, Aaron and Nina had similar tastes in music. "Fruit Salad, Yummy, Yummy" was a song Miriam, Nina's mom, played to teach the students at Wings how to communicate their taste for their favorite fruit. Miriam was a progressive speech pathologist who structured her lessons around play, music, and interaction with neurotypical peers. Therapy sessions were structured around age-appropriate casual play guided by studies based on research pioneered by Dr. Pamela Wolfberg in collaboration with Dr. Adriana Schuler from San Francisco State University. These therapeutic interactions were called Integrated Play Groups.

Nina was the more experienced player, and Aaron, the novice player. She loved to pretend, making her dolls move around the plastic doll house while she made up stories. Aaron would sit next to Nina, seemingly disinterested in the activities in the doll house, but fully engaged with the music coming from the boom box. In his own way, he was fully participating in play. Dr. Wolfberg's work identifies parallel play as a natural way to begin coordinating social interaction around shared interests.

From a very young age children learn social skills through playful interactions—first with caregivers and later, with peers. In the Integrated Play Groups, Aaron began to engage with others in ways that were normally accepted. He sat next to Nina, rather than running away and finding solace in a corner of the room. Miriam taught us communication was more than spewing out words: it was about reciprocal interaction and mutual engagement that leads to authentic connection with another being.

From where we sat, we could clearly see The Wiggles move from one side of the stage to the other, in unison with the anxious energy coming from the children, who orbited the auditorium like buzzing bees. The mini beings moved to their own rhythm, aligned with the tempo of the larger flock. Nina swayed to the beat of the song "Riding in the Big Red Car," while Aaron sank deeper and deeper into his chair, his knees getting closer to his chin with every move Nina made. Aaron's energy was packaged differently than that of his neighbors. He had his own way of processing the sounds and information that bounced around him. Others interpreted his behavior as anti-social; what he was showing was an inability to relate and communicate his emotions.

During intermission, we wiggled our way through the bopping heads towards the patio, where we could hear each other again. Nina and Miriam stood in line at the snack bar while Aaron and I waited away from the crowd. Suddenly, Aaron held his fists up in front of his face and moved them as if he was milking a cow. I bent down to meet his eyes—he seemed intent on telling me something.

Nina came back holding a bag of corn chips for Aaron.

"Chug, chug, chugga chugga, big red car!" She started singing and jumping up and down to The Wiggles' song, moving her hands the same way Aaron was. Miriam looked at me, somewhat puzzled by their interaction.

"Aaron, do you want to sing the song?" Miriam asked as she knelt next to him. Aaron's face became somber, and he moved away from her.

"Do you want to go to the car?" I asked. This was my way of asking him if he was ready to leave. Aaron walked towards the exit, and I followed.

"I guess he's all done with The Wiggles," Miriam said to Nina.

"But it's not over!" Nina said, and stomped her foot.

"It's Okay. Aaron is all done and wants to go home," Miriam said.

"But it's not time to go," Nina said, and started to cry. She looked confused by the smile on her mom's face.

"We can stay and see the rest of the show," Miriam said as they waved to us and headed back to the auditorium.

Miriam and I looked at each other from afar, knowing Aaron had made a quantum leap. He had made an intentional request and without knowing it, Nina had been his translator.

Aaron's pattern of communication began to evolve as he got older. Nina was able to understand his intentions effortlessly as she interpreted his peculiar sign language and connected it with a scene we had all witnessed a few minutes before: The Wiggles moving through the stage in the big red car. Of course, he had intentions— I just was not aware of them. I was looking for verbal signs familiar to me rather than seeking his intention by tuning into the slightest gestures, sounds, or even the direction of his gaze. We began to communicate in a very subtle way as I became aware of his energetic messages, which required me to listen from a deeper place. I began to understand what my teacher meant by being still and how differently we take in the world when we develop a quiet space within ourselves. Children have a more immediate access to this place that speaks the truth within themselves. I got a glimpse of what my teacher meant by being aware of being aware.

A View from the Kitchen Table

Over the years, as I gathered with other parents in their homes, we cried and shared our experiences at the kitchen table, skipping over idle talk and going right for the details that would lead to strategies to help our children thrive. Safety came to take on a broader meaning. I began to feel safe with those who were able to share their raw emotions and trusted me with their most vulnerable thoughts.

As I entered the kitchen in the home of a bereaved parent, her daughter rocked on the floor, flipping a string in front of her face as she made animalistic sounds.

"I don't know if I should stop her or let her continue," the mother said anxiously.

"Hi, Blessy!" I said, and knelt next to her.

"Say, 'Hi!'" the mother said as she grabbed the string away from the girl. I felt my heart sink, remembering my own agitation around Aaron when he would not respond to my request.

On the refrigerator door, Polaroid pictures of a milk carton, an apple, a plate, a car, a garbage pail, and a park bench gave a glimpse of the child's day. The countertop was riddled with the familiar: a visual timer shaped like a red disc that counted down time, plastic bottles full of supplements, and the usual clipboard with a list of to-dos.

Visits to the home were part of the Wings admission process. As the director of this specialized school, an unplanned role in the field of education, I was unaware of what was appropriate. This intimate view into the daily life of another family was humbling.

Suddenly I found myself leading a mission with a single focus—to improve the quality of the lives of the children who attended the school. The mission was broad and important. We adopted an approach not common in the public school system: rather than teaching children to become functional adults in a world that did not understand them, we first worked to understand the children and meet them where they were. Then we allowed them to lead us in developing a plan that would guide the curriculum and their unique individual education plan (IEP).

A digital calendar helped me organize the meetings and interviews that were part of the admission process. Kitchen conversations were real and revealed more about the parents than the child. Teachers continued the process at the school as they observed the child interact with other children and teachers in the classroom. The education team then decided if the child was admitted to the school or not. The question came down to: could this child benefit from being in our intensively focused classroom, or would she be better in an inclusive environment?

Wings teachers were sensitive sleuths, looking for signs that would open a window into the child's internal world. Everyone was a teacher, including each child. Questions were the beginning of the process: what made the long-legged girl run away from the classroom, swiftly and determinedly? Where was she going? What attracted the boy to the evergreen bush—was it the color, texture, or smell of the leaves that drew him close? What made the girl lick the chalk from the blackboard? Every day was one of discovery, leading to more unanswered questions—until the window opened and the child stepped out, even for a second.

The stories at the kitchen table were different from my own, but the sadness, frustration, and fear about the child's future were shared. Birthdays were sad reminders of unmet milestones.

"I never thought birthdays would bring so much sadness," one mother said as she placed a piece of her son's birthday cake on the table. "He just stared at the birthday candles," she recounted. "'Make a wish!' everyone shouted around the table," she continued as tears began to flow.

"Just blow like this," his younger brother had said as he blew out the candles.

At a visit with another mother, she recalled the day when, attempting to get her daughter's attention, she broke a plate on the kitchen floor. When her three-year-old daughter sat undisturbed, she knew there was something wrong.

There were rare times when both the mom and dad sat with me, sharing a cup of tea and cookies, each taking a turn, eager to tell me how well April behaved when the teacher gave her the attention she demanded. The most uncomfortable interviews were with parents on the brink of divorce. The mother would blame the absent father for their son's behavior, and the father would share how the chaos drove him away.

One parent described his son as "mildly autistic." It was a glimpse of how he wanted to see his son.

"He's really smart. Can read and count," the father said. The hundreds of parents I met over the years were mourning for the child they thought they had and lost to autism. They were looking for some way to get them back; they wanted a "normal" child.

"He's doing great in the classroom, he just needs a little help on the playground," a mother said proudly. "He just needs a bit more help and he'll catch up." She pleaded to get her son admitted to our school.

"Once he's caught up, he can go back to public school," another mother said. Sadness and worry filled the room. "He's getting older and needs to be back in a regular school." She leaned forward in her chair. "Oh, I need to tell you this. He only eats white rice and pears, peeled, with every seed removed. Otherwise, he won't eat," she continued. "Will that be a problem?"

"For his health?" I asked.

"No! For the school," she said.

There are reasons behind every idiosyncratic behavior. Barry Prizant writes, "Autism isn't an illness. It's a different way of being human... We need a way to understand them and then change what we do."

During the early years, I was so focused on my son's behavior that I didn't even consider my own. With the help of my life coach, I gradually became more aware of my internal world. I then began to make space to understand Aaron and my own responses to his behavior.

Philosophers, sages, and mystics have been pondering the human condition for thousands of years. Autism was recognized only in the first part of the twentieth century. We have much to learn about this other way of being human.

"I don't like the way the teacher talks to Andrew. He gets upset at him when Andrew doesn't understand what he's asking," a mother said.

"He's so smart if he were only given a chance!" Tears begin to flow.

"They're not teaching him anything at school. They're just babysitting him. He needs to be reading and writing. He's falling behind," the father said to me about his son, who could not sit still or focus on the teacher.

Parents were anxious and eager to give their child a chance in a caring environment, knowing there was so much more to their child than their arbitrary behavior. I connected to other parents in the ways they responded to the threat of seeing their children living encased in an autistic body. Trust was necessary, but so difficult to access.

"How do I know this school will be around in two years?" a skeptical mother asked.

"My son is a student at this school," is all I said. Her shoulders dropped and she smiled coyly. At that moment, I felt my responsibility to this mother and her son. I had stepped into a new place in this new world of autism. She wouldn't take just any answer. A confident mother bear, protecting her son. We needed each other. She and I became good friends, and her son was a student for the remainder of his school years.

There were parents I never met. Rusty, the only child we admitted whose parents were absent, was a bright and complex boy. I shed tears as I reviewed the notes: to protect her other children, his mother was forced to place him in a group home at the young age of eight. Did she even know if her son would ever return home? I saw myself in her shoes because I had asked myself: am I capable of mothering my own son? I had known I could not do it alone.

I visited Rusty in a special education school. A bright-eyed boy with red hair, his thin legs moved nervously in his baggy shorts. He looked down at me from the top of a desk moved to the corner of the classroom, which overlooked the playground.

"Get down!" a stocky man, who was assigned as his one-on-one aide, shouted. Rusty ignored the command as he looked down at me.

Our eyes met as he offered me his clenched fist. I moved my hand to meet his and he placed a marble in my palm. As I looked at what he'd placed in my hand, he jumped down and ran towards the playground. His aide ran after him. I wondered if this was a distracting gesture or a gesture of peace.

"He's a runner," the teacher said. We watched the man chase the small, wiry kid across the cement play area. "And a fence-climber. He looks for the right opportunity to take off. It's hard to find aides who can keep up with him," she continued.

After much thought, we decided to admit him to Wings. This was going to pose a new challenge for the teachers. I often thought about his mother. How did she feel when she read a report from the school about her son's life? He was doing math problems and writing complete sentences, yet he was never able to restrain himself long enough to stop from bolting towards an open space. What was he running towards or away from? Was he looking for something? A response from the teachers? An emotional jolt? What was going on inside that wiry body?

"Are you ready to do math?" the teacher asked. He was silent as he looked towards the open window.

"You are so good at it. Give it a try," she insisted. He didn't move. When she walked away, he looked at the worksheet on the desk for a moment, then walked towards the door that led to the playground.

"It's time for math," the teacher said as she followed him. He ran towards the play structure, climbed up the ladder and looked down at the teacher as his feet dangled above her. A half hour or so later, he came into the classroom, took the sheet and a pencil, and completed the worksheet. He then tore it up before the teacher had a chance to see it. When she pieced the worksheet together, he had completed every problem correctly.

Dear Dr. Schuler

I didn't go to your funeral. What could I say to your daughters, friends, and colleagues who gathered to honor your life? Words didn't always flow with ease for me, especially when my emotions were fully engaged. What was present for me when I heard of your passing was how you brought an understanding about connection built on respect, and insight into the uniqueness of individuals on the autism spectrum.

I'll begin by talking about play. You were known to embrace a *joie de vivre*. I can only guess your inner child was what connected you to the work that made a difference in the lives of so many children with autism. I remember when I first reached out to you, curious about the connection between play and autism. Play as an intervention for autism—seriously? As I became more familiar with your studies, it became clear: play, social interaction, and communication have a common thread.

After several unreturned calls and voice messages, you finally responded to a note I sent to your office at San Francisco State. At that time, in 1999, you were supervising interns working on their credentials as special education teachers. Aaron was seven. After being home-schooled for several years and fully included in a kindergarten classroom, we were ready to give special education a try. In this classroom, he needed a "shadow aide," and I didn't trust the school to provide him with one, so I set out to find my own. What I wanted was someone who would do more than shadow him around the classroom. I trusted your methods and sought out one of your students, who would be a respectful and caring guide for

Aaron. The young woman who arrived at our door was the right person Aaron needed at that stage of his growth.

Because it's difficult for Aaron to understand social rules, he learned his own coping strategies, which were not always understood by those around him. Neurotypical children pick up social cues as they grow up and interact with their caregivers and peers. Autism causes a disruption in the way children understand and read the world. Play is a safe way for children to learn from their peers and to learn the social dynamics that will be evident in the larger world. Aaron's behavior showed us how he was taking care of himself, by withdrawing from social settings he did not know how to deal with—smart boy. Like many parents of non-verbal children, I thought speech would be his way into a social environment. What I learned from you was that communication precedes speech; without communicative intent, speech becomes a string of rambles and may give those who are not familiar with autistic tendencies the false impression that an individual is communicating with a clear intention. Communication is an interaction between two or more individuals. Something else I learned from you: in the interactions which happen during play, a bridge is formed between the players that, when crossed, leads to a mutual understanding of the other person's intents.

Remember Aaron? When you met him, his vocabulary was sparse, maybe fifty or so words. When he did speak, words simply spewed out without intention—demands or requests—he named what he saw in front of him or what was in his mind. Now, at the age of twenty-eight, his communication skills have evolved; he makes himself clear even without having formal, verbal speech. He's very creative. With gestures, written words in books, and brief messages he types on his small machine, he connects with others by giving them the chance to ask him yes/no questions.

Words don't need to be a part of play. In fact, meaningful play often happens when children are jumping from one square to another, swinging their arms above their head, making silly faces, yelling at one another in the pool, growling like a tiger, or building imaginary cities in the sand. Who am I to tell you? You were the one who brought this insight to the attention of many educators.

You introduced me to one of your students, who "wanted to make a difference in your son's life." This young student not only bonded and connected with Aaron, but soon became a respected teacher and mentor to others who were learning how to connect and teach children on the spectrum. As an international student, she struggled with similar issues in communicating with others and understood the frustration Aaron faced when around others who had processing challenges. She was the right person at the right time for Aaron, and you brought your wisdom and insight at the right time for many educators, who learned that learning is not linear and can happen in joyful engagement with another human being.

In commemorating your life, I would mention how you influenced a group of professionals to start a school using a new model of teaching—one that guides students towards learning rather than trying to shape their behavior by responding to short-term reactions. You encouraged us to enhance communication in functional settings. I can still hear your voice getting louder and more animated as you spoke: "If you are teaching them the word 'cut,' then go to the kitchen and cut an apple!" You not only advocated interaction and play with neurotypical peers—you called them Expert Players—but also encouraged a process to teach neurotypical peers how they could engage those who could not play naturally. These groups were called Integrated Play Groups, and helped neurotypical children learn how to be compassionate, listen, and observe, while having fun and behaving naturally. Play is a skill that comes naturally to neurotypical children, but not to those with autism. Through play, cause and effect happen in rapid sequence, so learning happens quickly. You taught me this through your work.

As I spoke about you, I would probably digress, like you were known to do, with stories of our meetings at a coastal brewery, where we planned the school you helped name: Wings. You inspired teachers and therapists to meet the students where they were, to listen and observe. Observation was not limited to students; it also applied to themselves. Each student was a source of knowledge and a mirror for the teachers. The child guided their own unique lesson plan. Students were the source of information to the educators and to those of us who were ready to listen. Our lessons as educators were informed by patience, listening and observing the child's behavior. "Behavior is communication" was a common phrase we heard from you. After twenty years, the school continues to serve many with autism.

I remember the time you came to observe Joslin, the intern you introduced to our family. She became a teacher at Wings. As you observed Joslin from the back of the room, she rolled around on a small stool, swiveling from child to child, responding to their communicative intent.

"I see you are really excited, Barbara," she said to the girl who was jumping up and down from her chair and pulling on a rubber chewy dangling from her clenched teeth. Without missing a beat, she turned to Aaron and said, "Wow, you are waiting patiently for your favorite song." Then, a second later, to the boy who was walking towards his lunch box, she called, "Adam, in thirty minutes we will all sit down and have a snack together," and showed him a timer with a thirty-minute mark clearly visible as she walked him back to his chair. The children were learning how to regulate their bodies and emotions and to change their behavior. They were communicating without using words. You left the classroom quietly, not wanting to interrupt. The note you left for Joslin remained taped over her desk: A masterful circle session. Like a symphony, you guided the children. Bravo.

From you, I learned that communication is all about listening and responding. Like me, many parents are eager to hear their children talk and hear their voice, without realizing words without meaning could become another conundrum to be untangled. Communication is emotional energy moving through a silent bridge between people. Words, gestures, facial expressions, and emotions are powerful transmitters of ideas and meaning. Only by quieting our own inner thoughts can we truly listen to what is coming across that bridge. This is true for all humans, not just autistic individuals.

As I write this, in 2022, you'd see signs of a pandemic. Children sit six feet apart in classrooms, keeping each other safe from the virus. Even before the pandemic, Integrated Play Groups were disappearing from classrooms. Schools are emphasizing academic progress, and test scores have become more important than play. I would sadly inform you that the Expert Players are almost extinguished. It takes effort to find a child who would be willing to sit next to another and pretend to be a pirate or an astronaut going on a mission to Pluto, or create a city from wooden blocks.

Standardized testing has made it nearly impossible for special education teachers to collaborate with regular education teachers and form Integrated Play Groups in their classrooms. You may say the pandemic offers a perfect opportunity for neurotypical siblings to play with their autistic brothers and sisters at home—well, not always.

We no longer speak with each other but at each other. Communication with emoji-like symbols is a common practice. They are like the icons used in PECS (Picture Exchange Communication System). If you were to drop into our neighborhoods, you would think the world had embraced the needs of autistic people. Look closer at the face of the boy walking down the street, chin against his chest, eyes glued to a screen, totally in his own world, ignoring the person walking next to him: no, that's not an autistic boy; that's an average neurotypical boy.

I remember you teaching Aaron how to use PECS by giving his partner a card with an icon; the partner received it and then responded to his request. Much of this interaction has been digitized and conceptualized by high-tech applications. These apps are efficient, visually stimulating, and even allow for customized voices, but they haven't improved communication; in some ways, I think they have moved us a few steps back. The pandemic has taught us the importance of person-to-person interaction and how crucial it is to our emotional well-being.

We miss you, Adriana. We'll remember you through your work, and your questions about our connectedness will continue to deepen our appreciation of our basic human capacities: our ability to dream and to create, to be curious about what is possible, and to communicate and connect with each other in ways that are not always obvious. By interacting with each other through play you reminded us of our common human thread: the need for connection.

Unrestrained Exchange

On an ordinary day with my unordinary family, in 2006, the onset of puberty came thundering into our world. We headed out to the shopping center early so we could avoid crowds. Aaron unbuckled his seatbelt, picked up a shoebox full of family pictures, and ran out the back car door, his thick, black hair visibly leading the way to the front door of the mall. He was short for his age, like his grandfather—under four feet tall. His little belly was beginning to show signs of oncoming puberty.

"Wait for Mama," I called out. The fear of losing sight of him was ever-present after the scary moment we'd endured just a few months before. Unnoticed, he'd walked out of the house, entranced by the music coming from his iPod, which he held close to his ear. Fortunately, a neighbor had spotted him walking barefoot down the middle of a busy street and called the police. After that incident, I affixed name tags to his clothes and bought an intrusive and impractical GPS device, which he took out of his pocket as soon as he felt the weight of it. Only when he was within sight did I feel a slight sense of ease.

Sherman followed close behind me.

"We'll be at Crate and Barrel," I shouted.

"Do you have your phone?" he yelled back. I held my cell phone above my head so he could see it and placed it in my back pocket. Aaron had other plans and headed for the Disney Store. I had been in the small store many times—it was an enclosed space and somewhat safe. I could now take a deep breath.

I always had a sense of impending doom when I was out with Aaron. I didn't know how he was going to react to the sounds of a baby crying, the sudden bark of a dog, or a person screaming. I looked for opportunities to observe him from afar so I could gauge his behavior. This gave me clues about how he would react when and if I was not around to intervene.

The large window gave me a clear view of the inside of the store. His attention was fixed on a screen playing a scene from The Lion King. He was so engaged in the music he didn't seem to notice my absence.

My mother had been diagnosed with Parkinsonism in 2004, and she had begun to spend less time at our home with Aaron. He began to join Sherman and me during our weekend errands, which gave us an opportunity to observe Aaron interact with others outside his structured classroom and safe home life. I was cognizant of the importance of unstructured social interactions and saw the outings as important. I was vigilant when we were out in public, remembering the police incident after which Sherman was ready to place locks on every door.

"We need to teach him to tell us when he wants to go outside!" I said, objecting to Sherman's response to the incident. This became a source of some of our loudest arguments: how much freedom to give him and how to protect him from harm.

We planned our activities consciously, creating safe and open environments as much as possible—both so Aaron could gain self-confidence and we could gain trust in him.

I stood outside the Disney Store and positioned myself where I had a clear view of Aaron as he stood in front of the movie screen. There I could watch him while I called my mother, as I did every morning. My father answered the phone.

"This woman does not want to talk today," he said in a frustrated voice. The symptoms of Parkinsonism had progressed to where she could no longer speak when asked to.

"Don't talk to her that way! She can't help it," I shouted back at him. Memories surfaced of the days when Aaron had begun to lose the few words he knew, when he was just two. First, he'd stuttered—then there'd been silence. Mother was following the same progression.

"She needs to try harder!" His voice grew louder. I tried to stay calm as I reminded myself that her illness also had an impact on him. Father didn't know how to help her.

Mother had begun to fall more frequently and scratches on the side of the car door caused reason for concern, until my father took her license away. Glassware and dishes disappeared from our cupboard, and it was clear mother needed care herself. Father became her primary caregiver.

For a moment, I became so engaged in the conversation with Father that I lost track of Aaron inside the store. I rushed in and saw him sitting on the carpet with a Buzz Lightyear doll next to his ear.

"It's time to go. Let's go look for Papa," I said abruptly and yanked the toy out of his hand, still feeling the emotions from the conversation I had just had with my father. Aaron followed the doll with his eyes as I placed it back on the shelf. A few seconds later as we stepped out of the Disney Store, I felt his fingernails dig into my arm. The box of family photographs flew into the air and photos scattered on the floor. I panicked but tried to regain my composure as I walked, his hands grabbing at my arm, scratching with all his might. Heads turned as I walked towards the front door. Aaron pulled at my sleeve with one hand and grabbed my sweater with the other, grunting like an angry monster.

"Do you need help?" a stranger asked. I couldn't answer back. I just kept walking.

Our hands and fingers intertwined like spiders engaged in a wrestling match. I moved my hands and tried to keep his sharp nails from tearing my skin further.

"Is he having a seizure?" someone asked as a crowd formed around us.

Aaron's long, agile fingers continued to wrestle with mine, every groan and twist of his torso positioning him for a stronger hold on my arm, my chest—he grabbed for any exposed piece of flesh. I tried to calm myself with a quick breath.

"Aaron, it's all right, it's all right, let's count, one…two…three," I said to him in the calmest voice available to me. The rhythm of counting sometimes calmed him; this time it did nothing but exacerbate his anger.

A young woman approached us, trying to help.

"Grab my cell phone in my back pocket," I yelled towards her. She took the phone from my pocket, not knowing what to do.

"Three…four…seven," I dictated Sherman's cellphone number as she entered it and placed the phone next to my ear.

"Where are you?" he asked. He could hear me struggling.

"By the front entrance," I said.

As the call ended, I noticed a tall, burly man in uniform walk toward us. He calmly took hold of Aaron's arms and placed them above his head. Aaron's fingers surrendered and suddenly he calmed down.

A minute later a fire truck pulled up in front of the mall, followed by a police car.

"Shit," I whispered under my breath.

"What's going on?" a young officer asked. I was relieved to see Sherman running towards us. He responded to the officer, anticipating what had just happened.

"We should take him in, you know," the officer growled. I wrapped my arms around Aaron and let Sherman take over.

"He's autistic and gets easily overwhelmed," Sherman said to the officer.

"I need to file a report...who's going to give me the information?" the officer asked.

"What do you need to know?" Sherman asked calmly.

I took the opportunity to walk slowly away from the crowd as I held tightly to Aaron's hand. For a moment, the pain from the scratches disappeared; all I wanted was to leave the scene. Sherman stayed behind with the police officer.

We drove home in silence. I felt numbed by the events of the afternoon. Anger, pain, relief, compassion, fear, gratitude—All were present. The pulsating sting on my arms and fingers reminded me I was alive.

A year after this experience in the mall, Aaron experienced his first grand mal seizure.

Hell's Gate

Several months after the incident at the mall, we found ourselves bodysurfing and playing under the sun in Kauai. Aaron was unusually quiet and withdrawn. Maybe it was the water, the sun, the heat. Before going to bed that evening, we took a walk around the neighborhood where we had rented a beach house. Aaron fell quickly asleep in the room next to ours. Around midnight, I woke up to Sherman's voice.

"HELP!"

I rushed in and found Aaron on the floor, his body shaking violently.

"What happened?" I asked.

"I think he's having a seizure," he said.

Aaron's body jerked to a steady rhythm for what seemed an eternity, but was actually only about a minute. He caught his breath as if he had just finished running a fifty-yard dash. His eyes were listless, looking up at me without engagement. He began shivering. I placed a blanket over his small body and held him. I felt numb, not knowing what to do.

The thought of driving in the dark on the windy, two-lane road to Lihue to find a hospital—this wasn't a wise option. Sherman and I looked at each other worriedly for a few minutes but decided to wait. It wasn't long after the seizure that Aaron fell into a deep sleep. I kept vigil all night, waiting for another seizure, constantly watching the clock and holding tight to a phone. It was 6:00 a.m. when I called our doctor in California.

Dr. Travor assured me there was nothing we could do to prevent more seizures.

"Hang in there, and come home as soon as you can," he said in a calm voice. Aaron slept most of the day following the seizure. I stayed close to him, monitoring his breath, anxious, not knowing what to expect. We left on the next available flight back to California.

This new medical emergency took us on another wild journey. I was not fully prepared for the treatment of what was a comorbidity. Epilepsy is common in about forty percent of individuals with autism. The following months were heavy with fear, confusion, unanswered questions. Aaron began to have convulsions almost daily, sometimes several a day—some were very mild and only caused him to stop in the middle of an activity as if pondering a deep question. Then he'd snap out of it and continue what he was doing. There were also many strong convulsions, which would result in his body stiffening and suddenly dropping to the ground. These months were pure hell as we continuously feared a worsening condition and didn't know how we would treat this new medical condition or who would help us. His primary doctor sent us to a neurologist, not realizing there are neurologists who specialized in treating epilepsy called epileptologists. I found this out years later, after attending a seminar on new treatments for epilepsy.

We thought finding a neurologist familiar with the sensitivities of those with autism was most important. We were turned away from one office after another because Aaron hadn't had a twenty-four-hour electroencephalogram (EEG), which was needed to isolate the location of the seizures. The EEG was a simple procedure most people could endure without much discomfort. For Aaron, having electrodes strapped to his scalp for more than a few minutes was highly uncomfortable; he would not tolerate it.

"Can't you talk to him and tell him how important this is?" the intake nurse asked.

"I can do that, but you don't understand. He has autism," I said, trying to stay as calm as possible.

"I'm sorry, but that is the protocol. You can practice at home and call us later." I heard this over and over.

I didn't give up hope in the search for a physician who specialized in working with children with autism. Maybe she would be more understanding of the quandary we faced. We obtained an appointment with Dr. Bello, who examined Aaron.

"I must admit, I don't have any experience with individuals with autism," he said on our first visit. He was able to place a few electrodes on Aaron's scalp and look for unusual activity for several minutes. "I don't see anything unusual, but we need to monitor him for a longer period," he said, looking disappointed.

"What about sedating him?" I asked.

"That would impact the onset of a seizure and be counter-productive," he responded.

Then began an education about epilepsy: anti-epileptic drugs (AEDs) and their side effects, absent seizures, convulsions, auras, unusual behavior, and more I did not know.

One of the neurologists suggested that if we obtained a functional MRI (fMRI) at Stanford, maybe a seizure could be observed. As we parked the car at Stanford Children's Hospital, Aaron began to have a seizure. We proceeded with the fMRI. As expected, there were no signs of abnormal activity.

More hurdles presented themselves when it was time to prescribe medication. We continued to schedule EEGs, hoping a charming nurse could persuade Aaron to keep the electrodes on his scalp. One doctor suggested we admit him to a hospital in Sacramento and try for a longer period of time.

"We have some very skilled and sensitive nurses at the hospital," the neurologist said, who himself had a son with autism. "If they can't do it, then I don't know who can." He sounded optimistic. We checked into the hospital a day later, hopeful we could obtain the needed EEG. Unfortunately, the charming nurse could not persuade Aaron to keep the electrodes on for more than ten minutes. We left the hospital disappointed and defeated.

The seizures were becoming more frequent, and my anxiety continued to become more intense. Frequent convulsions drained Aaron's energy, and his behavior became more and more uncontrollable.

The search continued for a doctor who could be creative with her approach. But we kept hearing the same message:

"We need this to record the activity in his brain for at least twenty-four hours," a nurse said with a look of disappointment.

"And what if there is no seizure activity?" I asked.

"Then we'll need to try again," she said.

This was the most positive response we could expect. We were going to continue trying, again and again. It was a test of wills, patience, and persistence.

Finally, we found a neurologist who was willing to prescribe a medication without an EEG. At the entrance to his office was a poster with hundreds of AEDs.

"How do you know which medication is best for Aaron?" I asked.

"Well, it's a shot in the dark. We need to try something and hope it works. Something is better than nothing," he said in a sharp tone.

What about the severe effects of the recommended AEDs, ranging from dizziness to abnormalities of platelet counts and liver function? Many of the drugs required regular blood tests to monitor the effect on the liver. Aaron could tolerate an electrode on his scalp for only a few seconds; how could we safely perform a blood draw every few months?

"We need to try something!" Sherman said to me. So began an experimental phase of AEDs.

We met a doctor at Sutter Health who was willing to test medications with us and closely monitor Aaron's response. Aaron had reached the age many had warned me about: puberty. His body was changing, and so was his behavior. We couldn't predict anything. Acts of aggression were more frequent and, even with medication, the seizures continued. It took several visits and many questions to educate us about medications that could possibly make a difference. Nothing was sure. I wanted some thread of certainty; there was nothing to hang on to. The doctor listened to our concerns and answered every question with a thoughtful response. This was what we needed most—to be heard. We felt comfortable with her and began to engage in a process of trial and error.

After tweaking several medications, we settled on a combination of Keppra and Lamictal. We observed a brief but optimistic change in the frequency of Aaron's seizures. Rather than daily seizures, he was having them every two to three days. It was a brief relief. But the side effects of Keppra led to more aggression, and soon we gave it up.

The predictions came true. His teen years were hellish.

"I don't know how long we can take this. What will happen when we're older?" Sherman asked. Aggressive episodes led to physical restraints or quick avoidance, which required more stamina from both Sherman and me.

"Let's stay healthy and strong," I said, somewhat jokingly. It was not an option not to, and we both began to take our exercise routine more seriously.

These were challenging years for us at home as well as at school. Teachers developed detailed behavior plans so we would be consistent in addressing Aaron's behavior at home and school. We had to find ways to physically protect ourselves from the scratches to our hands and arms which resulted from an aggressive episode. He was getting stronger and older, while we were just getting older.

As Aaron reached his nineteenth birthday, the classroom staff could no longer deal with his behavior. Through his behavior he was telling us that he'd had it at school. Some days he would refuse to get out of the car. His school years ended with a graduation ceremony at Wings. It was a sad day when Aaron said goodbye to his teachers and friends, with whom he'd shared classrooms over the past eleven years.

Robert, a young man who was patient and calm, became his in-home teacher.

"What now?" I asked him.

"Aaron's been told what to do at school for so many years, why don't we let him tell us how he wants to spend his time?" Robert answered, with a certainty that made me trust his suggestion.

So began Aaron's time at home as we waited for him to tell us what he wanted to do during the day. We gave him choices: go to the beach or the park, listen to music, watch a video, or many other activities that once had been favorite pastimes, but were limited at school. During the first months at home, he spent most of his time in his bedroom, looking at books. We made as few demands as possible. It was a trying time for me; I felt like we were wasting precious time when he could be learning to become an independent adult.

What we learned in those two years was that trust was more important than skills. Trust in himself and those around him. Slowly he began to show more initiative and to make requests. One of his favorite activities was to ride around in the car with no specific place in mind.

"Do you want to go left or right?" I'd ask as we drove around our neighborhood. He'd signal left and I'd follow.

"What about now?" I asked one day, when we reached a dead-end street. "Straight ahead?" We couldn't go straight. I questioned his decision as he pointed to the house in front of us. "You want to go to see who lives there?" I asked.

"Huh!" he nodded. That's when I began to follow the hints— he was trying to tell me something.

"Do you want to get out?" I asked, and followed him out of the car, not knowing where he'd want to go.

I followed his lead as he walked towards this stranger's home, determined to ring the doorbell. I intercepted his hand when I heard the sound coming from inside. I peeked through a half-open window and noticed a television set was on.

"Do you want to watch TV?" I asked.

"Huh!" he nodded.

"Okay, let's go home and you can watch there!" I said, and he followed me back to the car.

Curiosity led to more and more circles of communication. He asked, and I responded, sometimes leading us to places I could not expect, like the entrance to the Oakland Zoo.

We continued to try other medications and settled on what has been the longest-lasting combination of meds: Lamictal and Topomax. When his seizures did not stop, we tried a more invasive approach.

Tea Time

I've met hundreds of mothers like myself over the years. Each encounter was an education in the struggles between being competent as a mother, longing to free their child from the prison of autism, and letting them go into independent adulthood.

When the holiday season came, I'd often receive a generous invitation from a woman who wanted to share holiday tea with other mothers of autistic children. In her posh Palo Alto home, we'd share stories and gossip for hours. Chatter was around toileting, enzymes, new medications, schools that were better than the last, therapists who charged inordinate amounts, district directors who had given in to parent's demands, classroom teachers who were angels, and the weight gain of their teenage sons—each story outdid the last, with brief talk about a promotion, travel plans, work projects, new books, or new exercise routines in between.

As the years passed, the conversations changed to locks on doors, overnight camps, Zoloft versus Abilify, sleepless nights, seizures, masturbating in the wrong places, night sweats, death, and divorce.

"Who is Billy going to live with?" one woman asked.

"We're both moving out and leaving him in the house. We'll take turns and take care of him, of course."

"Wow, that can get expensive," another remarked.

"Not as expensive as the therapist and the list of medications she was prescribing," another said as those around her burst out in laughter. Most of us had shared a part of her experience at one time in our lives.

There we were, a group of overworked mothers, slogging through common experiences and comparing grievances that filled us with gratitude, tears, remorse, and concerns about our children's future—doubtful and hopeful all in one experience shared by many.

Several mothers gathered around a buffet table after a memorial service for a friend, mother, and advocate for families and children with autism.

"Did you know she lost two of her sons a few years ago?" one mother asked.

"The only one left is Patrick, the one that needed her most; that's not fair," another said. What is fair, anyway?

Stories shared by mothers older than I, who had experienced the pain of their children's passing, fueled anxiety within me. I grew more bewildered with thoughts about how I would deal with the unavoidable truth of my own loss of faculties and eventual death, which would keep me from being my son's most competent care-giver. The idealism that had been part of my younger self began to crumble. Once, I was certain a charmed life would continue: from the days when I was a single woman with dreams of travel and a bohemian life as an artist, to a perfect motherhood with a supportive husband and family. I had yet to process the pain my grandmother and mother had lived through. The pain was not becoming real in my own life. But slowly, the universal pain all mothers share was revealed. I could never have imagined my own experience would become the granular material that fueled my inner work and self-discovery.

One Breath at a Time

Dreams often faded as I opened my eyes and woke up. No matter how much I tried to remember the stories, as soon as light entered my eyes, they crawled back under the rock of my unconscious. Once I knew Aaron was well cared for at Wings, my sleep became less interrupted by my worries, and I was able to relax. Six hours of sleep was all I needed. My dreams became more vivid, and I began to recall more details. In them lingered worries about how to handle the seizures and how to research medications with the least number of side effects. And always, worries about Aaron's future hung over me like a nebulous blob. I'd scour the dreams for clues about where to take the next step.

Aaron was becoming more curious about academics; reading, numbers, and puzzles began to interest him. His teachers focused on this curiosity and built on his interests. He seemed happy and more engaged in the world around him.

"Who is happy?" his teacher asked as she held up a book with a picture of a boy and a girl showing different emotions. Aaron was still learning how to point, so she would take his hand and point at the picture that matched his expression.

Babies learn to point early in their development. This is a sign of engagement with another person and the outside world. Neurotypical children begin to engage with others and the world around them at the age of eighteen months, a crucial step in communication and speech development—it's part of joint attention. Pointing is engaged attention. Aaron did not point to objects until he was about eight years old.

During a visit to the grocery store, he casually walked up to a Coke machine and stared at it.

"What is it?" I asked, somewhat puzzled at the intensity of his gaze. He then pointed at the Coke.

"Coke! You want a Coke?" I asked excitedly. I knew he'd tried this drink at his abuelito's house; they knew we did not approve of the sugary drink. Of course, I rewarded him with the Coke and was thrilled with this major milestone.

At school, he was learning how to identify emotions—his own and those of others.

"Is the boy happy?" teacher Amy asked, after waiting patiently for a response. She exaggerated a sad expression on her face. Aaron did not like to hear the word "No," and Amy was sensitive to the emotional response to the word. She guided his hand and pointed to the girl on the page. "Yes, the girl is happy!" She smiled effusively and Aaron did the same.

His face lit up as he took her hand and placed it on the book, wanting more. This was a new way of learning—being praised for what he could do, not reprimanded for what he could not.

New skills began to emerge. He learned to ride a bike, swim, and roller skate, and he became increasingly open to new experiences. He was spelling simple words on the keypad, and his love of books intensified; he began to read. I felt there was more space between his life and mine, and I could take time for myself.

With the help of a life coach, I began to learn about my personality patterns and the automatic coping strategies I defaulted to as a way to be in the world. It was a new way of looking at myself. I began to see I had a choice in how I viewed my life situation.

One of the most revealing lessons came when I recognized my need to scan for all the possible things that could go wrong during my day. Each morning I'd wake up to a visual image of how I imagined my day would evolve. I'd predict the events that would take place during a meeting with a school director and then set up a strategy for how to deal with this imagined scenario. Then I'd move to the next imagined threat. It seemed like a natural way to address life's situations, like I was being proactive. The strategy made me feel safe, but kept me from being present with what actually happened during the day. When everything went well, I attributed it to my cleverness and predictability. When there were problems, my anxiety level increased and I asked myself, what did I miss? My hyper-vigilance was taking me away from what I wanted: to feel safe and to keep conflict far away from my family and me.

Several years of coaching, meditation, and yoga practice helped me become more aware of my habitual personality patterns. What was once unconscious hyper-vigilance now became a choice. Before going into a meeting with a school director, which could become contentious, I breathed and took time to calm myself. I was often surprised by how meetings turned out.

Something else began to happen during this time of self-reflection: I became more aware of my body's responses to stress. When I sensed my throat tighten and my voice become softer as I spoke, I knew I needed to breathe and take a break from the situation. The demands did not diminish, but my way of handling difficult situations changed everything.

"No phone calls after six!" Sherman demanded one evening. I was so self-consumed that I had not paid attention to how my actions were affecting Sherman.

One day, my calendar was free of evening meetings—no big decisions to make or problems to solve. What a relief! My mother had left dinner simmering on the stove: oxtail stew, one of our favorites. I was about to start the rice cooker when I heard a crashing sound coming from the office above the kitchen. I ran to see what had happened, and as I opened the door, there stood Sherman. He was visibly angry, his chest was moving in and out, his fists clenched, and his lips pursed. Around him on the floor were the remains of a broken cup and scattered papers. He looked straight at me.

"I'm tired of being ignored as if I don't exist. All you care about is Aaron! What am I, a piece of meat?" Each word came at me like a thunderous blow. Caught off guard, I launched into self-defense. How could I not focus on Aaron? Didn't he understand the severity of the situation? What else could I do? Then I considered how I had been avoiding seeing what Sherman was experiencing? Maybe I didn't want to acknowledge his pain. That evening we slept on opposite sides of the bed.

When I met with Roxanne, my life coach, soon after the incident, I was ready to tell her about the event and be validated for my actions.

We began the session in the usual way, by "settling in"—sitting across from each other in matching high wingback chairs. With eyes closed, hands on my thighs, I leaned against a cushion that held my back erect. She reminded me to place both feet on the ground, take a deep breath, and relax. I had been introduced to meditation when I first began my sessions with her and still felt ill at ease in silence.

During the next fifteen minutes or so, she guided me through a process that has changed my life. With a calm voice, she led me through several minutes of self-observation: watching my thoughts as they arose and letting them go without judgment. That was the hardest part, letting go of judging myself; I wanted to get rid of my thoughts and just be in silence. Thoughts came in like a movie, cluttering my mental space. Mental activity is part of being human; how could I not know this? Through this process of meditation, I learned how to observe my mental activity and, in the process, open up space for mental clarity. This seems like a simple concept now, but then it was a revelation. I sat in silence as she spoke softly, new-age music playing in the background.

"Allow thoughts to come in and let them leave out the back door. When another thought comes in, watch it enter your awareness, and then let it go. Don't let it take you with it. Your thoughts are visitors—they come in and they go out. No judgment. Just watch the thoughts. Breathe."

Between the words, moments of silence followed. At first, I was uneasy just sitting and watching my thoughts, but after a few moments, I began to feel relaxed, at ease.

"When you're ready, come back into the room, and open your eyes," she said.

I settled into the chair, ready to begin recounting my story.

As I recalled the events of the evening, I began to feel the anger I encountered that evening with Sherman. I noticed my voice become softer. She interrupted me.

"What's happening in your body?"

What? In my body? How does that have anything to do with what I'm telling you?

"What's happening inside?" she asked.

Inside me?

I continued with my story, and she gently interrupted me again.

"What sensations are present in your body?" she asked.

That question—what did it mean?

"I don't know," I said, somewhat embarrassed.

"Let's explore it, shall we?" she asked. I had no idea what that meant, but went along as she guided the process. One question followed the next.

We began to explore what was happening internally for me in that moment. She would take me back to what was happening in my body. I became aware of how my body responded to the event.

"What are you sensing right now?" she asked.

"My throat is tight," I responded.

"Tight," she repeated. "Breathe into the tightness," she said, and breathed with me as I sensed the tightness. I didn't know what that meant, but I followed her and breathed slowly, in and out, staying with the discomfort inside my throat. After a few breaths, she asked me another unexpected question.

"What is the quality of the sensation?"

I didn't know how to answer, and she followed with another question as I sat motionlessly.

"Is there texture to the sensation?" she asked. "Coarse, rough, soft?" she clarified.

"Ummmmm," I made something up. "Coarse," I said, and felt even more uncomfortable.

"Is there a temperature? Warm, cool, maybe nothing at all?" she asked.

"I don't sense any temperature," I said.

"Stay with the sensation, is that okay?" she asked, and continued to be very much with me as I felt even more uneasy with the questions.

"Yeah," I said reluctantly. We sat in silence. I became more conscious of my breath and the tightness in my throat.

"Stay with it," she insisted. I continued to breathe and, for the first time, I felt the sensations that had been with me but never acknowledged.

"What's happening?" she asked.

"I'm feeling something in my chest," I said.

"Is there movement?" she asked.

"Yes. It feels as if it's swirling, like a dry tumbleweed inside, moving around."

"Dry," she repeated, and took a breath along with me. In slow motion, I sat with the sensation of a tumbleweed twirling inside as the discomfort intensified.

"Stay with it," she said.

That is the last thing I want to do. I want this to be over. What's the use? This is ridiculous. I came to tell her about Sherman's anger. Is he right? Am I being inconsiderate? Now I'm just being uncomfortable in my own skin. Wait, I'm feeling my own skin, my inside. This is new—something I've not done before. I'm experiencing sensations not through my thoughts, my head. Have I been ignoring my body? There's something here that feels foreign, but at the same time, real.

Minutes felt like hours.

"What's happening right now?" she asked.

I could not explain what was happening.

"I'm scared!" I said as tears began to well.

"Breathe," she said. "It's okay to be scared. Can you stay with it, the emotion, for a bit longer?" she asked.

As I noticed my breath, my emotions intensified.

"What do you want to do now?" she asked.

"I just want to cry." I placed my head in my hands and allowed the weight on my chest to push the tears out.

"Give the tears permission to come. It's okay," she said, and we sat together until there were no more tears and I let myself feel the release.

We never talked about the broken glass or the reason why Sherman was so upset. I expected to analyze the event. Instead, Roxanne's questions led me to experience my internal landscape for the first time. It was about the experience, without judgment, analysis, or answers. I witnessed myself for a few minutes, something I had never allowed myself to do.

The drive home was blissful. I was in a daze. Something inside me had changed. I wanted to allow whatever it was to continue. I took a detour to the Pulgas Water Temple, where the waters from the Hetch Hetchy Valley in northern Yosemite, empty into the reservoir. The park was desolate except for a couple of sunbathers sprawled on the lawn overlooking the reflecting pool. I passed them as they embraced. I kept my eyes on the Corinthian columns that stood around the opening, where the waters from the northern glaciers gushed through to the Crystal Springs Reservoir. I looked down the well-shaped opening and felt a cold breeze from the movement of the glacial waters. Drops of moisture splashed onto my face. Behind me, yew trees swayed in unison as the gentle summer wind reminded me life is not stagnant, but ever-moving, like thoughts that are visitors only for a moment. I had found an intimate stranger inside me. One that could echo my external experiences with real, live emotions and sensations that moved through my body.

The years passed quickly as Aaron became a teenager. He continued to grow at his own pace, communicating in his own way. He was heading into manhood, reaching out to a world that now made a bit more sense to him. I was on a different path, learning to go inward and listen to my body for clues and messages that could not be analyzed, predicted, or formed in my head.

I was beginning to understand the meaning of the sign at the entrance to Roxanne's office: Expect Something Wonderful to Happen.

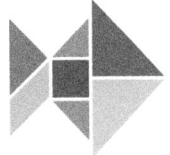

PART 4
A Way Home

"The individual is essentially the collective,
and society is the creation of the individual.
The individual and society are interrelated, are they not?
They are not separate."

—*Total Freedom*,
J. Krishnamurti

Nothing to Fix

Being a mother is like being on the battlefront: the first to meet the bullets, and the first to see glory.

It was 4:32 a.m. when the sound of the commuter train rattled our bedroom window, and I faced that December morning in 2012. The winter solstice was two days away and the end of the world, as my Mayan ancestors had predicted, was closer to becoming a headline. I reached over to feel Sherman's warm feet for just a few more minutes before stepping onto the hardwood floor. Sunrise yoga, a centering practice recommended by Roxanne, had become part of my morning ritual. On alternating days, I headed to the gym to focus on my heart so I could stay away from another heart attack scare.

Aaron was still asleep at 9:00 a.m., oblivious to the surgery scheduled for later that morning. Robert was rather unpunctual; the thought increased my anxiety level as I began to prepare for the day ahead. He was in charge of Aaron, as he has been for the past two years as Aaron's caretaker, teacher, and friend. I briefed him on the morning regimen: nothing to drink or eat, loose clothes. Make sure you bring: talking machine, laptop, book, backpack, hand brace, meds—check, check, check. We discussed our strategy. I would text him twenty minutes before Aaron was to enter surgery; they must be ready to move swiftly. I had timed the drive to the surgery room: twenty minutes, door to door.

Sherman followed me out the door. We kissed goodbye, as we did every morning before he left for the office. "I'll see you at the hospital around eleven, after I answer a few emails," he said.

I stopped at the Kaffeehaus for my first cup of coffee. Aaron and Robert were regulars there, not for the coffee but for the social scene with a familiar crowd. This was part of creating a social environment for Aaron. Seeing him around others gave me some hope that, someday, he would learn how to socialize on his own.

As I drove past the exit to my parent's house, I imagined my mother saying, "What if he's hungry? It's cold—don't forget his jacket!" My father would chime in: What if they don't understand him? Don't forget to tell them how he threw up after the anesthesia last time! Mother tended to caress Aaron's black hair while calling him pobrecito. This comment made my stomach hurt and my back tighten. It brought up a feeling of pity for him, and maybe for me—feelings of incompetency that I rejected. These emotions became part of my sessions with Roxanne as I explored the underlying beliefs that drove my coping mechanisms. I tightened my grip on the steering wheel as I merged towards Highway 280. I had planned the morning carefully. I was on schedule.

Detailed preparations were part of our family routine. Aaron was anxious in unfamiliar places, so I tried to make transitions as smooth as possible, planning the most minor details. As I began to understand my own behavior, I realized these preparations were more for me than for Aaron.

When I arrived at the waiting room, every chair was occupied. One or two people were tapping on their cellphones, while others looked at the clock or stared out the window on that windy morning.

Dr. Esperanza walked confidently towards me in his sky-blue scrubs, his brow showing the familiar glow of perspiration. But he walked past me to greet the gaze of a middle-aged man who looked at him with anticipation. My elbow tipped over a plastic Christmas tree on the corner of the desk as I reached for the paperwork from the attendant. The power of attorney was on top, followed by forms with details of Aaron's birth, medical conditions, and allergies. I reviewed carefully line by line: first, middle, and last name: check. Right shoulder arthroscopy: check. I glanced for instructions and made sure the right shoulder was clearly noted at every instance.

One last thread of doubt was removed. The information was accurate. As I handed the papers over to the receptionist, a woman came out from the side door and called Aaron's name. I had learned to appreciate efficiency because it reduced the angst that waiting produced for Aaron. We always found ways to fill the time to ease his anxiety. We prepared a social story, explaining in detail what to expect. He enjoyed when I read it out loud. Sometimes I'd write in long hand what was about to happen; he listened attentively as I read. I wondered why the movement of my hand over a blank piece of paper hypnotized him. Was it the shape of the letters, the sound of the pen on paper, or the meaning of the words? Even when the letters were illegible, he remained consumed, and followed the movement of the pen. I'd always keep a watchful eye for signs of tightness in his forehead or his front teeth hugging his lower lip.

I checked the clock and began to strategize how I was going to bide time until Aaron and Robert appeared. As the nurse came out and called his name, Aaron walked through the door and directly into the surgery room, where the nurse was waiting for him. I breathed with relief and followed him inside the prep room.

Sue, the admitting nurse, asked him if she could take his blood pressure. Before I could answer for him, he nodded, and she carefully wrapped the blue cuff twice around his upper arm.

"It's going to squeeze your arm, okay?" she said, and looked at his face. He nodded. "One hundred over sixty-five, very good," she said with a reassuring smile, and quickly ripped off the cuff. Dark-skinned women often brought a smile to his face, especially those with Asian features. Over the years, he'd learned to keep his distance from others, especially women. After years at school, at the age of nineteen, he came to understand the meaning of keeping boundaries. Eye contact was a sign of connection, and he used his wisely.

He took the paper robe in his left hand, never letting go of the laptop with his right. I was reminded of the surgery to install a vagus nerve stimulator on his left chest just two months before. He changed into the robe quickly and took a seat next to me, his thin hips squeezing between my thighs and the arm of the chair. He was consumed with his favorite show, Between the Lions. Just then the curtains parted. He stood up without hesitation and followed Sue, the nurse who had charmed him minutes before. His paper gown offered me a glimpse of his slender buttocks. Sue clapped and sang along with the song as they walked together into the operating room. I waved and blew him a kiss, his back towards me. He was on his own.

Sherman waited for me in the cafeteria. It was a cool and breezy morning as we both hugged our cups of warm tea between our hands.

"Two hours at least," he said, trying to bring some certainty to the moment.

"He went in happy," I assured him.

"He responds well to pretty women," I said, after I told him about Nurse Sue.

"These Nordic winds are going to last the rest of the week," he said. Sherman liked to look at the future for some signs of certainty. I looked ahead with unwavering optimism; this was a possible course that would reverse the pain Aaron had been through. My trust in Dr. Esperanza had grown over the years—he had been consistent and kind, making time for home visits when I texted him with another incident of a dislocated shoulder. Aaron's low muscle tone and constant seizures had destroyed the tissue in his right shoulder. My own doubts about the medical system made me postpone the decision to proceed with surgery.

"We need to operate on him. His shoulder is not going to heal on its own," said the doctor in a stern voice. Aaron was in pain, and we could not wait any longer.

Some things can be fixed. Broken tibias, gun-shot wounds, torn ligaments, even skin destroyed by fire. It seems pain is more acute when the fix is near. My doubts masked the pain Aaron and I were feeling. A fix seemed far away until I made the decision to schedule the operation.

I didn't want to look at the X-ray of his torn shoulder—his ligaments and pink tissue looked like crumpled wrapping paper, barely holding his humerus in place, battered by years of convulsions.

There was no way to fix the pain he had endured.

"At least I can fix this one," Dr. Esperanza said. His sweet smile was reassuring as he walked towards Sherman and me, ready to update us on the result of the surgery.

"All went well," is all I wanted to hear.

"This is the worst shoulder I have seen in my years of being a surgeon." His words cut through me like a sharp razor. I walked into the recovery room, relieved it was over and Aaron would soon be free from pain. His arm, bandaged and covered with gauze, made him look larger than his slight frame. Now he had two wounds. My heart broke as I looked at his chest.

"I can't fix my son's obsessions or his anxiety, but at least I can fix Aaron's arm," said Dr. Esperanza, placing his hand on my shoulder. We'd become friends over the years, connected by our children—Dr. Esperanza's son, who was Aaron's age, also had autism.

Pain had been a companion through many sleepless nights. Pain also comes with motherhood—a pain that can't be compared with any other flesh wound. It's felt in the heart, deep in the chamber, pulsating with each thought of the slightest discomfort my son may feel. It lingers until the smile comes and I know he is okay, at least for that moment, which is all we have.

A curtain separated the recovering patients from each other. Aaron's face was pale, his lips dry and chapped, his eyes half open. An oxygen sensor masked his finger, a needle covered by bandages was in his left wrist, his right arm was wrapped in a Darth Vader shoulder stabilizer. He couldn't move.

In my early twenties, I thought I could fix anything with a good intention, hard work, and perseverance. That's all I needed. Some of this belief was instilled by my grandmother, who prayed next to me before going to bed: keep us far away from the doctor's office, put rice and beans on the table, and yes, never let my parents miss a day of work. She believed if you didn't get what you asked for, you were not working hard enough. Her work ethic was strict and consistent; after all, she fed and dressed nine children and nursed a bedridden husband. I remember uniforms neatly folded and stacked in the corner of her sewing room. She always found a new way to make ends meet and keep food on the table for her children. If she could do that, I could fix anything. This was part of my belief system.

Autism is untreatable, yet individuals respond positively to treatment methods and therapies. Parents continue to hope for the miracle that will make their child walk away from the corner of the room and look into their eyes, jump in the air with unrestrained joy after catching a ball in the infield, or blush with embarrassment when the girl he's been eying gives him a kiss on the cheek. Treatment options are as unique as each person, with lesson plans that can only be developed by caregivers who listen to their children and to themselves. Once enrolled in this self-guided, unstructured program, parents are asked to stay the course and adjust the curriculum as they go along. There is no right or wrong way of parenting. We do our best by following the lessons lived through the complexities which show up as our children grow into adulthood.

After years of listening to reports in hours of meetings with deft therapists and medical professionals and looking for signs of behavior that resemble normalcy, some give up, leaving wounds in marriages and relationships. The clock starts ticking at the time of the diagnosis. Each birthday marks another milestone in time.

Birthdays don't need to be a sad acknowledgment of unmet milestones. They can be a celebration of another year of heroic effort by their child to understand the complexity of a world that doesn't understand him.

Get ready for puberty, we were told; it gets worse. And in adulthood, you better have a plan, a trust, and a mentor. Our family made it through puberty, with wounds and scars.

Aaron walked out of the recovery room and ignored the wheelchair the nurse was holding for him. My mind began to spin with details of his recovery and a worst-case scenario that could take us back to the surgery room. Days passed, each day his shoulder becoming stronger and more ready to tolerate the seizures, which continued.

The fix restored an illusion of order and health to Aaron's arm. I could now accept his other human frailties, as well as mine.

I've coped through life by anticipating what is next. This strategy has served as an anchor and provided me a false sense of security. Over the years I've come to allow a more powerful practice; one of setting intentions and trusting the mystery of what unfolds. When I choose to allow the unknown, I've been met by countless possibilities that shine through the smallest pinholes.

The Step You Don't Want to Take

I was five years old when I experienced fear. That's what I call her now, but I had no idea who she was that evening when I walked down a cobblestone street in the middle of a desolate pueblo near San Salvador, where I lived. I was walking next to my older cousin, Noy, whom I trusted.

"There she is," Noy said, looking towards a shadow walking toward us. The moving figure looked like an old, decrepit woman I had heard of many times before.

"*La Siguanaba!*" Noy said as I grabbed for her skirt. The old woman glanced at us before she was engulfed in the darkness of a *meson*, her dwelling place, which was as mysterious as the legend that followed her in.

Folktales resembling those of *La Siguanaba* can be found in many cultures. When I was growing up, this mythical character was part of the stories my caregivers told to scare me into becoming a compliant child. I was told *La Siguanaba* was an old woman with a hunchback and gourd-like abscesses between her chin and chest. The story went this way: during the evening she would scour the streets for mischievous children, whom she'd later drag into the woods and eat alive. I only half-believed the story until that evening, when I saw her in the flesh.

She looked like I'd imagined her: long, stringy hair; elongated face; dark, deep-seated eyes; and a hunched back that dwarfed most of her upper body. It was the growth protruding from her throat that took her humanity away and made her face and upper body monstrous. I stood paralyzed, shaking in fear, holding on to immature beliefs that were meant to keep me scared and dutiful to the demands of elders who could not find other ways to make me comply with their demands.

Fifty-some years later, I found myself in Taos, New Mexico, at the edge of the desert, joined by a group of fellow explorers of inner truth in a week-long retreat held at Mabel Dodge Luhan House, a few miles from the Taos Pueblo. I took this time consciously as mine, away from family and responsibilities, to explore my inner self. The open New Mexico sky and desert, dotted with pinyon trees, was a perfect place to settle into my interior self.

Whenever I had a free moment between talks that were meant to help us get closer to ourselves and understand the psychological structure of our inner territory, I walked the labyrinth and meditated. We were encouraged to bring the practice of presence to each moment as we walked and engaged with our fellow retreat participants. The practice took me from a conceptual understanding of this state to real experience in the moment. I began to notice a more intense connection with my surroundings. The autumn leaves revealed gradient shades of burnt sienna, and the air met me with more immediacy when I walked out into the chilly morning. It was an intense week of self-inquiry, punctuated by moments of discomfort.

Towards the end of the retreat, our group was led into a mystical and ecstatic experience by Belinda, a psychologist, teacher, and follower of the work of the cultural anthropologist Dr. Felicitas Goodman. The ritual was a doorway out of habitual life experiences to a place where we could let go of the limitations of ordinary consciousness and be in an alternate state of reality—another new experience for me.

The room where we met had thick walls. I felt like I was in a sanctuary where the other participants and I could experience a novel ritual. A stage was at the east side of the room, where nine-foot windows opened up to a majestic view of Taos Mountain, also known as the Sacred Mountain.

We stood in a circle as the sun began to set. The group had shared a meal in the communal living room, and comments on the delicious vegetarian dinner of mushroom soup and roasted vegetables were part of the conversations circling among us.

"Let's prepare ourselves," said Belinda as she lit a match and set afire a bundle of dry sage resting in a porcelain bowl. Smudging is part of ceremonies—a way of cleansing and purifying our souls to clear out our emotional clutter. Smoke engulfed the room, and the evening dimmed the inner space. Each person in the circle took the porcelain bowl and moved the smoke around their bodies to smudge themselves. The woman to my left held the bowl for me so I could scoop smoke with both hands and bathe myself with it. I then held the bowl for the man on my right. We went around the circle until all participants had cleansed themselves.

Belinda invited the spirits to join us as she stood in the middle of the circle with her arms open wide. She offered a pinch of cornmeal toward the four directions: east, north, west, and south, and then above, to Father Sky, and below, to Mother Earth. She then gently caressed a rattle she held in one hand with cornmeal and whispered, "Wake up, little sister."

We sat in silence for a few moments. Belinda demonstrated a posture or pose we were about to hold for fifteen minutes as she shook the rattle. The pose seemed simple: left hand cupped around our left knee, right hand on lap, both feet on the floor and tongue touching the lower lip. Eyes closed.

"When you hear the rattle, we will begin. The ritual will end when you no longer hear the sound. You can then move," Belinda said.

I felt my shoulders tighten, then took a deep breath and settled myself on the chair. Everyone around me looked calm. I wondered if I appeared the same, while inside I was feeling anxious, and curious. I closed my eyes and tried to be present to the sound of the rattle and the scent of burning sage permeating the room.

Since I was very young, I have been curious about ways of accessing a different level of consciousness. Having experienced a séance and hypnosis with my Uncle Sergio, I could not help but hold doubt about the séance experiences. I began to open to this new experience and allowed my whole self to engage in the ritual that was about to begin. I was aware of a state of consciousness that lies dormant during our ordinary day, and I wanted to access that part of me.

Belinda explained that the sound of the rattle, similar to the drum, stimulates the nervous system and opens one up to a trance-like state. The rhythmic sound of the rattle began to fill the room, and I felt my heart join in the rhythm. Slowly my anxiety quelled, and I was able to move into the experience. With my eyes closed, I saw the image of my Abuela Esther, standing in the north corner of the room. She stood like I remembered her standing at the front of the church altar—erect like a soldier, waiting for orders from above. My other abuela, Mirtala, my father's mother, also appeared. I could see her leaning against the east wall, with her hands crossed in front of her tummy. Close to the bathroom stood my mother, an appropriate place for her to stand, practical as she was. Behind me, closest to the door leading to the courtyard, was my maternal great-grandmother, Ilaria. Aunt Rose was there, too, standing firm in the middle of the stage, facing the room as if she was about to conduct an orchestra. But where was my father? Somehow, I knew he was also in the room.

I saw him briefly; then he disappeared. These images were clear in my imagination as the rattle sounded in the background and I sat still, engaged in the pose.

Fifteen minutes passed quickly, and then the sound of the rattle faded into a long silence, until Belinda spoke.

"Continue to stay in the sacred space this evening. No talking until tomorrow morning, when we will meet again for our last day together," she said. The group moved ceremoniously, in silence, out the door.

I walked out and felt the cold, dry air of the evening touch my face. I had every intention to go to my room and continue to be in silence; instead, I walked out toward the driveway, which led out to a dark street, away from the main compound. I continued to walk. I didn't know where I was going, but something told me there was somewhere else I needed to be.

The sound of the gravel underfoot echoed the sound of the rattle I'd heard only minutes before. I was being guided by an uncontrollable force. All I could do was follow, one foot in front of the other. I passed a dimly lit sign announcing the entrance to Mabel Dodge Luhan House. I was being moved and had no control over it.

I kept walking, and under a streetlamp, I was moved to look back at the dim lights in the compound. I then continued past a large, blue dumpster jutting into the street. I remembered seeing it that morning when I had walked to the plaza.

The road disappeared in front of me behind a black curtain of darkness. There was just enough light for me to take a few steps toward an unknown destination. For a moment, a thought came to mind: no one knows where I am, or where I'm going. I felt alone, and at the same time, guided by a familiar companion. My senses were heightened, and I heard a television playing a beer commercial. I turned into a dark alley and continued to walk.

From afar, unintelligible voices echoed from an open field. The alley led to a park, a gathering place for the local community. I remembered that during a morning walk, I had passed by the park, where several women sat around a picnic table drinking from brown paper bags. I paused in the darkness and sensed the silhouette of an iron gate in front of me. I felt calm and alert as I walked and heard the rustling of dry leaves under my feet. Suddenly I felt a flash of fear. Should I turn around? Am I safe? Where am I going?

I sensed my father's presence and heard a voice: Take the next step. Then you'll know what to do. It was my father's voice. This time I could not ignore it, although many times I had. I continued walking in the darkness.

I came to a tall iron gate—the entrance to the Kit Carson cemetery. I walked through the gate with confidence and, after a few steps, came to the location of two graves, faintly outlined by the backdrop of street lights. Darkness blurred the names on the gravestones, and I stood there for a few seconds. Then I began to weep. I allowed myself to feel unrecognizable emotions that had no meaning. All I could do was let tears flow. Is this a dream?

I'm not sure how much time passed until I felt settled. I then picked up a few leaves from the nearby sycamore tree and stuffed them in my coat pocket, dried my tears, and retraced my steps back to the house.

I was glad we had been given directions to stay in silence that evening. When I walked into my room, I waved to my roommate, picked up my journal, and wrote down the experience in silence until I fell asleep.

The next morning, I rifled through my coat pocket and found the dry leaves from the sycamore tree. It wasn't a dream.

Years later, I returned to the cemetery and retraced my steps. The graves I had visited were those of Kit Carson and his third wife, Josefa. Carson was an illiterate man who gave up an education to learn a trade. He was a fur trapper, a guide, an Indian agent, a soldier. Born in Missouri in 1809, he died a month after Josefa in Colorado in 1868. Taos became his home base after long expeditions and hunting adventures from east to west. The house where he lived is now a museum on Main Street.

My father's life followed a similar thread. After high school, he joined his uncle as an apprentice and became a skillful carpenter. He furnished the modest home where he lived with my Abuela Mirtala and his sister, Rose. He was also an adventurer, leaving his country of birth in 1963 to settle in California. He didn't know where he was going or what was ahead for him or his family, but he took the next step—one that changed my life.

I've visited Taos many times since that retreat. The dirt roads, Taos Mountain, and soft, rounded adobe homes, along with the aromatic coffee houses, art galleries, and Taos Pueblo fill me with memories of the evening my ancestors visited me. They had all departed this earth. Since that evening, I've called on my father's spirit and held on to the message he left for me: Take the next step, and you will know what to do.

Letting Go

The word surrender makes me uncomfortable, especially as a mother of a son with autism. But when I hear the word "death," I fall apart. I come face to face with the most painful death I could imagine—that of my son. Why would I want to imagine my own son's death? I'll let you into my inner world.

When Aaron began to experience seizures at the onset of puberty, I asked the neurologist how dangerous they were. She answered unexpectedly:

"People don't die from seizures."

"Most of the fatalities result from an unexpected accident while having a seizure—falling, drowning, having an accident while operating a machine or driving a car. The seizure is rarely the cause of death."

I was somewhat relieved. It gave me the illusion that I could keep Aaron safe if I planned and was cautious. Her answer allowed me to wrap my fear in a self-woven wool blanket, an illusion of control.

Over the years, I have experienced unthinkable events, grieving friends who died in accidents or have lost a child to an event like the one the doctor predicted. The unforgettable afternoon when I experienced the grief and pain of a father who had lost his son in his backyard pool after he experienced a seizure was almost unbearable. It could easily have been Aaron in that pool.

These words are difficult to write. I believe that what I imagine can come true. Over the years, I've come to accept and allow the discomfort of this possibility. When the thought comes, I take a breath and feel into the sensations that arise. Sensing into my body's sensations has been a practice that has taken me to a deeper awareness of my capacity to stay with what is real and present at the moment.

I've been close by when Aaron had a near-fatal fall during a seizure, missing a sharp edge, knowing his *abuelos* were looking after him and had kept him from a threat to his life. Then, after a fall, I'd touch his head, shoulder, arm, looking for blood. Then, as soon as he'd caught his breath, I'd check for cuts and rush to the refrigerator to get ice and take the next breath. I'd made it a point to never be out of reach when he was in a bathtub or swimming pool, near a knife or sharp corners. I constantly scanned his environment for danger.

Yet there have been moments of surrender. Those moments came after years of continuous seizures and staying with the internal pain that is part of being a mother.

There were other ways I'd surrendered, such as when Aaron experienced overnight camp without a caregiver who knew his every wish.

It was time for me to let go of my fear of not always being close to him and for him to experience his capacity for independence and enjoy being in nature with friends his age. He could gaze at the stars overhead, sing silly songs around a campfire, and sleep in a cabin with other men his age. But, most importantly, he could be away from Mom and Dad. As a teen, I'd envied those who had spent their summers at camp. I could only imagine what it was like. My parents did not have the means to pay for the luxury, so I never asked.

I finally gathered the courage and came across a camp for adults with special needs called Via West. Aaron was already twenty, and I thought it was time for him to experience being away from home, at least for a few days.

A weekend at a beautiful retreat-like camp in the woods without me to look after him. We had protected him, as had his care-givers and teachers, who had come to know him well. They could interpret his facial expressions, sign language, eating habits, vocal sounds, mannerisms—they knew him and understood his world. He was never alone.

The day of the camp arrived after I had filled out pages of forms, requests from doctors and therapists, details of eating habits, behaviors, medications, medical references, nightly rituals, and communication. The twenty-page questionnaire gave me some comfort; it asked for every detail we could want to provide. I knew he would be safe at the camp. The volunteers were loving and engaged with him as if they knew him. Via West had been operating for over twenty years, and had a tradition and reputation of safety and care for those they served.

The campsite was nestled in the Cupertino foothills, next to the Stevens Creek County Park. A windy road lined with ancient oak trees against a backdrop of redwoods led to the site. Deer slowed cars, which stopped to let them drink from a flowing creek. I walked with Aaron towards the front desk, a paper with a list of questions in hand. How do you keep campers safe when outdoors in open and wooded surroundings? What if he wanders off? Who watches the campers at night? The camp director had an answer to every question.

I waved goodbye and walked calmly to the car holding Sher-man's hand. Aaron rolled his well-stocked suitcase behind him, and his counselor carried his backpack and pillow under his arm. They disappeared into the cabin where he would sleep in a bunkhouse with twenty or so men his age.

Via West gave individuals like Aaron an experience that supported their independence. The counselor was used to seeing mothers like me.

"Don't worry, we'll take good care of Aaron," the woman at the welcome desk said.

"There's a nurse on site all weekend," she assured me.

"Do you want us to call if he has a seizure?" she asked.

"Yes, please," I said as I checked the number on the form to make sure it was accurate.

After years of camp experiences, Aaron has gained confidence in himself. He has made friends and established his communication style with the camp staff and participants. I was always surprised to read the comments on the forms he brought home with him:

He likes to cook.

He enjoyed coloring and drawing.

He and Tom had a good time at the baseball game.

I no longer ask him if he wants to go to Via West; instead, it has become a place where he can be himself with his friends, who treat him like another regular guy.

That first weekend was when I finally allowed myself to let him go. I expected my phone to ring any minute, asking me to pick him up. He made it through the weekend without me. What a sad relief. Slowly, he was moving away from me.

"Did you like camp?" I asked. He buckled himself in the back seat and nodded firmly. It was undeniable: Yes. I took a deep breath, and we drove home. The smell of redwoods came in through the open window. Aaron was tired and calm. I was happy, and my heart was open as we looked out the window. We were both changed by this experience.

While Aaron was becoming more independent, I was more at ease knowing he was out in the world without me. I knew deep inside that he was not going to be able to live on his own, that he would be interdependent with others.

Separation from my family in El Salvador was a jolt away from a tradition. One where there was an underlying presumption that aging was an experience we shared with our family and closest friends. When the time came, we would care for each other. But, as I took in the American way of being, family security thinned into doubt. A nagging fear kept me awake at night with the question: what would happen when Sherman and I were no longer on this earth taking care of Aaron's every need?

Every parent of an adult with autism arrives at this place later rather than sooner: what will happen when I'm gone?

Abuela

At 8:00 a.m.

she walked

into the kitchen, where she cooked

all day.

That evening

her apron hung behind the kitchen door

where she left it

after she said

goodbye.

When I'm Gone

"Who's going to take care of him when I'm gone?" These were the last words I heard my father say, a few days before he passed. His voice was quivering, and his brown eyes had lost their luster. I wondered if he could even see me, but he knew I was the one standing next to his bed.

My mother had passed in 2009, two years before, on the same bed they shared for fifty-six years. His cheeks were sunken, and stubble covered most of his face. It had been months since he could get out of bed on his own, his heels bruised from touching the same spot on the bed—signs of the damage diabetes had done to his body. Aaron, his first-born grandson, was the love of his life. A month after this conversation, in December 2011, he left us. His last words hung in limbo over me.

Although the question seemed to address a time far into the future, I began to worry. Who was going to take care of Aaron when both Sherman and I were gone? I was creeping into my sixtieth year. Of course, deep down I was aware that life is temporary and I could die at any moment. But when I did die, who else was capable? The question began to work me at a deep level.

I have a confession. Almost every morning, before getting out of bed, I visualize a list of my trusted circle of friends. This ritual was part of an unconscious habit of scanning for threats around me. The list contained allies who would help me fight off inner dragons, friends whom I could trust in case of an emergency, and my dear extended family, for whom I'm grateful. As I got older, my family elders had been departing. Even friends my age had passed. As a family elder, I now sit at the end of the holiday dinner table. The trust offered some solace, but without the love behind it, it was just a piece of paper backed up by an illusion of security.

"The executor can even be the trust department at your local bank," our attorney said. How sad would that be?

My father had raised more and more questions, which had become impossible to ignore. We now had Aaron's future to plan, not just our own. Who would ultimately be responsible for Aaron's health, and where would he live? Who would live with him?

Looking back at the people who had been in Aaron's life and the love that had surrounded him—family, friends, caregivers, teachers, health professionals—I took comfort in knowing that Aaron has a natural way of attracting people who come to love him. I had no need to worry, but I did.

Preparation was the only way I could stop worrying; prepare a plan, create a community around him, document his social structure, and let those who cared for him know about his network of support. It was like preparing for a fire—practicing a fire drill so everyone else knows what to do when the fire comes. As I've grown older, I have come to trust this deeper knowing that I, and Aaron, are held by a power greater than all of us.

Where will he live? That seemed to be the most practical place to start. Even though a building does not make a home, it does provide a sense of security. We began to scout out locations in the Bay Area where Aaron could live the rest of his life. Ironically, we settled in Windsor, a small enclave in Northern California. It had all the appeal of a cozy town. Rather than having a plaza, the center of the town was accentuated by the Town Green, a large, open area where people gathered, played, and enjoyed weekend concerts. We began a development project with other parents, that would house eight other adults with developmental disabilities. It was a parent-driven project.

Three years into development, as we neared the design phase of the project, it all fell apart. We learned several valuable lessons from this endeavor. The most important one was that a community of individuals, not a group of buildings, formed the foundation of any housing community. Unfortunately, I didn't learn about the work of Otto Scharmer until years after our failed attempt. In his book, The Essentials of Theory U, Scharmer expands on the cultivation of social fields. He compares social fields to the soil of an organization: "Attention must be given to the quality of relationships between individuals, teams, and institutions that give rise to collective behavior and practical results."

Great communities don't just emerge from the good intentions of the participants. Underneath the examples of housing developments across the country intended for individuals with disabilities must be conscious work done to strengthen the social fields. We looked ahead to the end result, but glossed over the cultivation of the social field of the future of Aaron's home. We failed to ask this important question: how do you maintain an open, honest, and thriving community of parents and caregivers as you develop the housing component of the project?

One positive outcome of our project was that we found our retirement community and Aaron's future home. We settled in Sebastopol, the town that welcomed my father in 1963 and was a jumping-off point for our lives in the U.S. In this farming community, the social field had rich soil. We were called to maintain, enrich, and take care of the fertile soil for it to continue to provide a nurturing home for Aaron in the future.

So, what was left but surrender? Not giving up but giving it up. Letting go of what I feared and my limited view of what was possible.

Gone Fishing

"Your mother wants to go fishing." I heard my father's voice on the other side of the phone. Another time he would have laughed at her request, saying how ridiculous she was. This time he was different.

"What? Are you sure she said that?" I asked, holding the phone tightly against my ear.

"She won't say it again. But that's what she said!" my father replied.

"I'll be right there!" I hung up the phone and rushed to their house.

For years, Mother had called me every morning before going to church. Her questions were short and predictable:

How is Aaron?

Anything new?

I'll be there later to prepare his lunch.

When will you be home?

Then the calls stopped. Shortly after Mother was diagnosed with Parkinsonism, she began to fall, became forgetful, and was often confused. The neurologist explained and made sure I understood it was another form of Parkinson's, not a mild form like I suspected.

"But her hands don't shake," I said.

"The symptoms are slightly different, but the conditions are very similar," he assured me, somewhat irritated by my questions.

Mother was in her early seventies when the symptoms started. Loss of balance, stuttering, forgetting words, sudden blank stares, unexpected falls.

"It was a stupid fall. All of a sudden, I just fell backward for no reason at all," she said, still shaking, and with a concerned look on her face.

As the years passed, she began to limit her activities. Falls became more frequent. Dishes, cups, and glasses disappeared from our cupboards. Mile-long walks to church turned into short jaunts around the block, assisted by a caregiver. Her sewing machine and knitting needles remained untouched. Her once-admired, classic penmanship morphed into unrecognizable scribbles. Then her speech was compromised; she talked less and less, until she no longer said a word. She slipped away into a silent world.

I wondered if she had given up or just lost her ability to form words around her thoughts.

She wants to go fishing? The last time I saw her hold a fishing pole was when I was a teen and we sat around for hours on the shores of Lake Shasta, waiting for fish to bite.

I was just getting used to Aaron's silence. I wanted to hear her voice again, even if it was for an unreasonable request. I was hopeful.

She was sitting in her usual place, a La-Z-Boy in the family room. The news on Univision was blaring on the television screen. Her eyes were frozen, looking straight ahead, but away from the television—a look that had become familiar.

"So, you want to go fishing?" I asked her. I waited for a long time—I was used to waiting.

"Siii," she said in a low and tender voice. "Fish for you and Tia Marta," she then said in a clear, hurried tone. Marta was her older sister.

My mother's illness and a new way of life took on an energy of their own. My father was an unprepared caregiver and started showing signs of frustration and stress. He became angry and impatient when Mother could no longer speak in complete sentences.

"She can talk—if she tries hard enough," he'd say in front of her. Her eyes opened even wider when she heard his insensitive remarks and was unable to respond.

"Let her drive. It will give her more confidence," he continued.

"Are you crazy?!" I asked, as the argument spiraled into an emotional exchange.

Vivian, a newfound caregiver, wrapped Mother's sweater around her shoulders and dropped bottles of medication in her purse. We drove to Pacifica, a small town on the coast. I wasn't sure what would happen on that cold and foggy afternoon, but I wanted to comply with my mother's request, as I did whenever Aaron asked for something. It opened the channels of communication. Who knew what else she would say? I allowed the afternoon to flow without any expectations.

Mother seldom asked for anything for herself. Over time, she and Father developed a comfortable relationship: he made decisions, and she followed dutifully. They had been each other's first and only love, marrying as they entered adulthood. Like most couples, they argued bitterly and often, mostly around his drinking and money. She'd often turn to her best friend and confidant, Mercedes, to unload until she, too, was struck with Parkinson's.

It was cold and overcast when we arrived at the docks that afternoon. The waves gently caressed the pier, where we could see men bundled up with blankets hunched over the side, waiting for a tug on the line. Mother gripped my arm and Vivian held her other one. She sauntered down the only place we could walk. She had a gentle, faraway look on her relaxed face.

When we reached the end of the pier, we stood and looked at the vast ocean. We walked for more than an hour, listening to the ocean slap against the posts of the piers under our feet. Seagulls flew overhead, almost brushing our heads as they dove for the scattered fish guts on wooden planks.

"There's a fish market down the street. Do you want to go?" I asked. She looked ahead in a silent stare and moved at a clumsy, steady pace as I guided her towards the car.

"What kind of fish would Marta like? Salmon or trout?" I held up my right and left palms in front of her face, as if to give her a high five.

This was the way I gave Aaron choices. After much practice, he learned the one he touched first was his choice.

She pointed at my right hand.

"Okay, salmon it is." And we headed for the fish market.

Her grip on my arm softened. For a moment, we were closer than we had been. For most of my life, our relationship had been distant. She kept her emotions close, seldom sharing them with me, but had some intense, private conversations with Mercedes.

Her life before she met my father was a mystery to me. She never wanted to talk about her childhood—only to share that it was difficult growing up as the youngest girl in a household full of men. Her older sisters left for the U.S. when they were young, leaving behind my grandmother, who depended on my mother to take care of her brothers and bedridden father. Then walking down the pier, I felt an unfamiliar closeness. Silence had lifted a veil between us. Maybe she understood a reality only Aaron experienced.

Over the next four years, Mother slowly slipped away from us, until she reached the place the doctor had warned about, the moment that signaled the end of her life—she lost her ability to swallow.

In the last days of her life, I played romantic ballads of her youth by her favorite trio, Los Panchos. I sat on her bed, and we shed tears together.

The last years with my mother were ones of surrendering to a life we had both experienced. We surrendered the resentment, anger, regret for a life I wished we could have had and stepped fully into our shared life. On a morning in May 2009, she slipped out of this world gently, as though the smoke of an extinguished candle filled the room with her memory.

Epilogue

I dream in the language of vibrant oranges, pulsing greens, and calming blues, creating a collage on the canvas of my subconscious. I sometimes speak in metaphors, using images to express my thoughts. Words don't always flow freely, but mental photographs flood my imagination with a clarity that I can't ignore.

As I dream of a future for Aaron, I envision him happy and confident living among others who are curious about his expressive language and open to the joy that he shares from his innocent soul.

When I ask my friends about their children, they often express pride in their career progress, newfound love, or family life, and usually there is an update on their travels. "And Aaron?" they ask. I tell them about his health, his new interest in Japanese DVDs, a history book that has been his companion for weeks, and the conversation he had with his art teacher over Zoom, all without using a commonly recognized word. I proudly tell them how engaged he is with Sherman and me, as well as those who share his space. Since 2020, during COVID-19, his social world has been Zoom classes and discussions with his peers. At times he participates, and at others, he remains silent. His teachers make sure that his presence is acknowledged, and he responds to being seen.

And where does he live? Others want to know. Independence is more important in our North American culture than in my ancestral home, where people age comfortably being interdependent with others. We've come to accept that Aaron will be living close to us until we die. In Sebastopol, California, we've begun to create a community where our family and caregivers will live in proximity while caring for each other's wellbeing. Aaron will be part of this community.

Our community has molded our world and created a foundation on which to stand, inspiring me to respond to the challenges we've faced. My family has given me traditions that have allowed me to remain in contact with the deepest part of my roots.

The questions that began when I became a mother continue to be present in my life and drive my passion as I engage with a broader community. I continue to place my attention on issues specific to Aaron's health and well-being. And on the larger world in which he will live.

Aaron is a shining light in our world, showing others the pureness of his intentions and the clarity of his soul. His presence makes all the difference in this world.

References

Books

Blake, Amanda. *Your Body is Your Brain.* Trokay Press, 2018.

Boone, Victoria M. *Positive Parenting for Autism: Powerful Strategies to Help Your Child Overcome Challenges and Thrive.* Althea Press, 2018.

Cutler, Eustacia. *A Thorn in My Pocket.* Future Horizons, 2016.

Gore, Belinda. *The Ecstatic Experience: Healing Postures for Spirit Journeys.* Bear & Company, 2009.

Grandin, Temple. *Thinking In Pictures: And Other Reports from My Life with Autism.* Doubleday, 1995.

Grandin, Temple, and Catherine Johnson. *Animals in Translation: Using the Mysteries of Autism to Decode Animal Behavior.* Harcourt, 2005.

Higashida, Naoki. *The Reason I Jump: The Inner Voice of a Thirteen-Year-Old Boy with Autism.* Translated by K.A. Yoshida and David Mitchell. Random House Publishing Group, 2016.

Howe-Murphy, Roxanne. *Deep Living with the Enneagram: Recovering Your True Nature.* Enneagram Press, Revised and Updated 2020.

Kaufman, Barry Neil. *Son-Rise: The Miracle Continues.* H J Kramer, 1994.

Kranowitz, Carol Stock. *The Out-of-Sync Child: Recognizing and Coping with Sensory Processing Disorder.* Skylight Press, 2005.

Mack, Arien, and Irvin Rock. *Inattentional Blindness.*
MIT Press, 2000.

Maurice, Catherine. *Let Me Hear Your Voice: A Family's Triumph Over Autism.* Ballantine Books, 1994.

Palmer, Parker J. *The Courage to Teach: Exploring the Inner Landscape of a Teacher's Life,* 20th Anniversary Edition. Jossey-Bass, 2017.

Prizant, Barry M. with Tom Fields-Meyer. *Uniquely Human: A Different Way of Seeing Autism.* Simon & Schuster, 2015.

Rimland, Bernard. *Infantile Autism: The Syndrome and Its Implications for a Neural Theory of Behavior.* First Printing, 1964. Jessica Kingsley Publishers, Second Edition, 2014.

Scharmer, C. Otto. *The Essentials of Theory U: Core Principles and Applications.* Berrett-Koehler Publishers, Inc., 2018.

Skinner, B. F. *Verbal Behavior.* Martino Fine Books, 2015.

Whyte, David. *The Three Marriages: Reimagining Work, Self and Relationship.* Riverhead Books, 2009.

Williams, Donna. *Nobody Nowhere: The Extraordinary Autobiography of an Autistic.* Times Books, 1992.

Winnicott, D. W. *Playing and Reality.* Routledge, 2005.

The Child, the Family, and the Outside World. Perseus Publishing, 1992.

Wolfberg, Pamela J. *Peer Play and the Autism Spectrum: The Art of Guiding Children's Socialization and Imagination.* Autism Asperger Publishing Co., 2003.

Websites

Autism Collective for Peer Socialization, Play and Imagination
http://wolfberg.com

Autism Treatment Center of America: The Son-Rise Program
for Autism
https://autismtreatmentcenter.org

Deep Living Lab
https://deeplivinglab.org

The Greenspan Floortime Approach
https://stanleygreenspan.com

Dr. Barry M. Prizant
http://barryprizant.com

Glossary

ABA
See "Applied Behavior Analysis"

Advocate
An advocate can provide coaching and strategies, advise about your and your child's rights, help with negotiations or presentations, review your child's IEP or 504 Plan, attend meetings with you, make recommendations of other service providers, and more. They may be a family friend, a teacher, an expert in a relevant field, a representative from a nonprofit organization, a consultant hired for assistance, or any other person you feel will best help you advance your child's rights to appropriate assistance. The advocate does not need to be an attorney, although they can be. Bottom line: You have the right to have an advocate assist and accompany you, assuring the best outcome for your child. The advocate may also serve as personal support for you.

Aide
A school-based paraprofessional who attends school with a child to support their learning in the classroom, including focus, impulse control, social and functional skills, following directions, and sometimes academics. They help the child become more independent over time in the school setting. Terms used in an academic environment are shadow aide, instructional aide, or instructional assistant.

Applied Behavior Analysis (ABA)
A practice for applying psychological principles in a systematic way to modify behavior. Board-certified behavior analysts may be part of a therapy team that supports an individual at home or at school. Dr. Ivar Lovaas, a behavioral psychologist, pioneered the application of the ABA approach to teach skills to children with autism. ABA is based on analyzing the antecedents, behaviors, and consequences of an individual's actions.

ASD
See "autism spectrum disorder"

Autism Spectrum Disorder (ASD)
A developmental disability that can cause significant social, communication, and behavioral challenges. The learning, thinking, and problem-solving abilities of people with ASD can range from gifted to severely challenged. The diagnosis of ASD now includes conditions that used to be diagnosed separately, including autistic disorder, pervasive developmental disorder not otherwise specified (PDD-NOS), and Asperger syndrome.

Circles of Communication
Relational Development Intervention (RDI) and Floortime Models use this communicative intent as a cornerstone of their therapeutic approach, which builds on emotional back-and-forth exchanges between an individual and caregiver that support development and social interaction.

Drill
An aspect of Discrete Trial Learning that involves highly intensive and repetitive components of tasks that facilitate learning specific behaviors.

Echolalia
Repetition of sounds or others' words, phrases, or sentences, either immediately, delayed, or used as self-talk. All children use repetition as part of learning language, with neurotypical children letting it go as they learn to use individual words to express their own thoughts. Echolalia continues for a longer time in children who have autism because they learn language differently, often in blocks of words that the child does not understand individually. Yet they often are forms of communication that can be built on as steps to flexible language.

Epilepsy
A chronic disorder that generates recurring epileptic seizures—sudden surges of electrical activity in the brain. Approximately one-third of people on the autism spectrum also have epilepsy. There are many different types of seizures, ranging from "absence seizures" that may look like staring spells to those that cause muscles to become weak or limp and those with muscle twitching or severe spasms.

Expert and Novice Players
These terms were used to describe both neurotypical and non-neurotypical players. Because the terms have been often misrepresented, they are no longer used.

FAPE
Free and Appropriate Public Education for students with disabilities - Section 504 of The Rehabilitation Act of 1973 protects the rights of students with disabilities to a "free appropriate public education," regardless of the nature or severity of the person's disability, under the Individuals with Disabilities Education Act (IDEA). An "appropriate education" is defined in the law as "services designed to meet the individual education needs of students with disabilities as adequately as the needs of non-disabled students are met," and may include related services such as speech therapy, occupational and physical therapy, and psychological counseling.

Floortime
Floortime is structured play therapy that builds on emotional and communication skills. Professionals, parents, guardians, and others can be play partners in various settings. Developed by Dr. Stanley Greenspan and Dr. Serena Weider, its focus is connecting with children through emotional relationships and joyful play.

Full Inclusion

Students with all abilities are integrated into the general education classrooms. Some preparation, accommodations, and special training for the teachers, students, and assistants that will be part of the classroom may be required for students to be fully included.

IDEA

Individuals with Disabilities Education Act is a federal law that was amended in 1997 to give civil rights to all children, including those with disabilities, to receive a "free appropriate public education (FAPE)" with related services that may be needed, in the "least restrictive environment (LRE)," individualized and appropriate to the child's needs.

IEP

Individualized Education Plan. The plan outlines a student's educational needs and the services that will be required to support those needs. Short-term and long-term goals are established by the IEP that include the parents, teachers, a school representative, administrators, therapists, and others that have knowledge of the student's needs. Ideally, the IEP creates a roadmap for how to support the student's successful development through their school years. The IEP is reviewed at least annually but may be reviewed with more frequency to ensure it continues to provide the support the student needs. The IEP is a legal document that is recognized by the school district where the student receives services.

Inattentional Blindness

A psychological phenomenon that occurs when an individual is focusing on one thing and fails to notice unexpected things entering his field of vision.

Joint Attention

The ability to share focus on an object or area with another person. Many people with autism have difficulty following someone's gaze or where someone may be pointing their finger. Developing joint attention skills is important for communication and learning language.

Mirroring

The brain's mirror-neuron system is activated when you subconsciously replicate another person's nonverbal signals as if you had initiated the same signals yourself. This may involve gestures, speech patterns, body positions, or other aspects. Normally, mirroring creates a feeling of connection and empathy with the person being mirrored. However, studies have indicated that the brain's mirror-neuron system is impaired in children with autism. Without the ability to imitate others' facial expressions and other nonverbal cues, neuroscientists believe that autism causes an incomprehension of others' emotions and makes social interactions confusing and difficult.

Neurotypical (also NT)

An abbreviation for "neurologically typical," widely used in the autism community for people who are not autistic, or more broadly, for people without developmental disorders.

Occupational Therapy

An occupational therapist utilizes assessments to develop, recover, or/and maintain meaningful activities of individuals so that they can live meaningful lives. For example, the therapist may identify sensory challenges such as dealing with bright lights, loud noises, or strong tastes or smells, and then develop strategies to help the individual self-regulate. They might help individuals develop boundaries, obtain appropriate social skills, gain independence in dressing or feeding themselves, or adapt to transitions in their routines.

One-on-One Therapy

Therapy can take place in groups or individually. One-on-one sessions are used to teach specific skills where the therapist can customize the experience to address the child's individual needs and give them extra support and attention.

Placement

A term used in education settings indicating the school location or site where a student will receive their education.

PECS

Picture Exchange Communication System. A system that allows a person without other clear communication abilities to express their needs and establish communication. Several studies have found that this method can help create a foundation for developing verbal language. PECS consists of six phases and begins by teaching an individual to give a single picture of a desired item or action to a "communicative partner" who immediately honors the exchange as a request. The system goes on to teach discrimination of pictures and how to put them together in sentences. In the more advanced phases, individuals are taught to use modifiers, answer questions, and comment.

Prompt

Prompts are stimuli used to provide an entry point into a main task. Prompts can be visual, spoken, or written. Resources that can be used as prompts include flashcards, realia, body language, facial expression, keywords, questions, and repeating errors.

Prompt Dependent

A person may be prompt-dependent when they do not take action on their own but wait for someone to tell them to take action. Since the goal for children with autism, as for all children, is to become as self-sufficient as possible, teachers or others learn to "fade" the prompt over time by extending the length of time before indicating a desired action. The intention is to give the child time to recognize the action to take without being told.

Section 504 Plan
Under Section 504 of the federal Rehabilitation Act, civil rights law declares that an individual cannot be discriminated against because of their disability. The 504 Plan outlines what supports and accommodations will be provided to the student by the school district, without cost. They are reviewed periodically according to need.

Sensory Regulation
The ability to attain, maintain, and change energy states, emotions, behaviors, and attention in ways that are socially acceptable and help achieve positive goals.

Speech Therapy
Speech therapy addresses verbal and non-verbal language and includes social communication. It may include help in strengthening the muscles in the mouth to speak more clearly. The role of speech therapy is to help individuals communicate more effectively and interact with others.

Stim
Shorthand for "self-stimulating behavior," sometimes called "stereotypic" behavior, often used as a self-calming and self-regulating behavior. Many neurotypical people use repetitive behaviors to calm stress, such as nail biting or tapping a pencil. Stims may be used to cope with anxiety or strong emotions, to manage sensitivities such as loud or high-pitched noise or bright light, or to calm in challenging or overwhelming situations.

Vagus Nerve Stimulator (VNS)
An FDA-approved VNS can be surgically implanted under the skin on the chest, with a wire threaded under the skin to the left vagus nerve. When triggered, the device sends electrical signals to the brain. Research into non-invasive vagus nerve devices is ongoing in Europe and the U.S.

Chapter Notes

ABOARD PAN AM FLIGHT 1206

El Salvador

The sixties were turbulent years in Central America. Fidel Castro's successful expulsion of Bautista in 1959 gave rise to fear that communism would take a stronghold in the Americas. The failed attempt by anti-Castro exiles in the 1961 invasion of the Bay of Pigs gave Castro more validity and increased the angst in Latin America. The tension continued with the Cuban Missile crisis in 1962 (https://www.history.com/topics/cold-war/cuban-missile-crisis).

The 1960s brought uncertainty to El Salvador. In 1960 a preemptive coup ousted the liberal president José María Lemus, fueling a slow-burning flame that led to a bloody civil war lasting through the seventies and eighties and leaving more than 75,000 people dead.

A painful but beautifully written book about the crisis in El Salvador is What You Have Heard Is True: A Memoir of Witness and Resistance, by the poet Carolyn Forché, published in 2019.

GATES OF HELL

Auguste Rodin's *Gates of Hell*

California's Stanford University, just south of San Francisco, is home to the largest collection of Auguste Rodin's sculptures outside of Paris (nearly 100 works). Some are displayed throughout the campus, but most are at the university's Cantor Arts Center.

FISH DREAMS

A number of studies have found a connection between a mother's recurring miscarriages and the long-term neurological health of a subsequent child. Surprisingly, older fathers may significantly influence spontaneous first-trimester miscarriages. Older age in both mothers and fathers increases the risk of autism in their child. But autistic children appear to be more likely to inherit risk variants from their fathers. These are questions I pondered but did not fully research to determine how this may have had an impact on Aaron.

Resources
Dorit Paz Levy, et al., "Maternal Recurrent Pregnancy Loss Is Associated with an Increased Risk for Long-Term Neurological Morbidity in Offspring," *Developmental Medicine & Child Neurology,* July 29, 2018.

Findings suggest a history of maternal recurrent pregnancy loss impacts the long-term neurological health of the offspring.
https://onlinelibrary.wiley.com/doi/full/10.1111/dmcn.13976

Riffat Jaleel and Ayesha Khan, "Paternal Factors in Spontaneous First Trimester Miscarriage," Pakistan Journal of Medical Sciences, May-June 2013, accessed at US National Library of Medicine, National Institutes of Health.

Findings concluded "paternal age beyond thirty-five years was found to be significantly related to first trimester spontaneous miscarriages."
https://www.ncbi.nlm.nih.gov/pmc/articles/PMC3809297/

Lisa A. Croen, et al., "Maternal and Paternal Age and Risk of Autism Spectrum Disorders," JAMA Pediatrics, April 2007.

A very large Kaiser Permanente study of children born in northern California 1995-1999, indicating the risk of autism increased significantly with each ten-year increase in both maternal and paternal age.
https://jamanetwork.com/journals/jamapediatrics/article-abstract/570033

Matt Warren, "Autistic Children May Inherit DNA Mutations from Their Fathers," *Science*, April 19, 2018.

Findings suggest that autistic children tended to inherit genetic risk variants in regulatory regions from their fathers, who tended to be non-autistic, and not from their mothers.
https://www.science.org/content/article/autistic-children-may-inherit-dna-mutations-their-fathers

THE ANGST BOX

Aaron was three when he was first diagnosed with autism in the mid-1990s.

Early childhood appears to offer the greatest possibility to enhance opportunities to supplement and expand abilities that are generally more challenging for children with autism than for most neuro-typical children. Therefore, significant research is finding ways to identify, at younger and younger ages, children who may have autism so that it can be addressed as early as possible. The hope is that early therapy, during the time when infants' and toddlers' brains are rapidly growing, developing, and have not yet solidified their circuitry, can minimize the difficulties.

At the same time, there is also hope for those with autism who are older. For example, Dr. Michael Merzenich, professor emeritus at the University of California-San Francisco and an eminent neuroscientist, has pioneered extensive research in the field of neuroplasticity. He found that, while infancy is a critical time for establishing neural processes, the brain continues to refine these processes even into adulthood. His vast creative work in brain science has led to innovative educational and cognitive training approaches, including Fast ForWord that has successfully helped children and older people with autism to read. He also led the development of Brain HQ, brain exercises to strengthen brain function, and the cochlear implant for addressing deafness.

Resources
Dr. Michael Merzenich, "About Brain Plasticity," On the Brain
https://www.onthebrain.com/brain-plasticity/

Why Early Intervention Is Important

In the past, children often were not diagnosed with autism until they were three or four years old, or even five, when they first went to school. But research has made it clear that intervention and therapies at as early an age as possible give a larger window to address an infant's or toddler's developmental weaknesses and bolster their strengths. Sometimes supportive therapy can even reduce the likelihood of an autism diagnosis at a later age, although that may not reduce the need for continuing therapies to focus on ongoing developmental challenges.

Today, clues that can recommend testing an infant for autism can become available even during pregnancy, and even more so within the first year of life. These allow parents and therapists to start helping children improve social abilities at very early stages of brain development, thus enhancing their potential for successfully navigating education and flourishing in the future.

Resources
Every autistic child or adult is different, with unique combinations of strengths and weaknesses that need attention. An important short video is:

Dr. Barry Prizant, "Tips for Parents Following an Autism Diagnosis (3 min)."
http://barryprizant.com/
tips-for-parents-following-an-autism-diagnosis/

Ian Sample/Science Editor, "Autism Therapy Aimed at Infants May Reduce Likelihood of Later Diagnosis," The Guardian, 20 Sept 2021.
https://www.theguardian.com/society/2021/sep/20/
autism-therapy-infants-study-social-development

Learning About Autism

It was very difficult to find helpful information about autism and how to navigate a successful path for my son and my family when Aaron was first diagnosed in the mid-1990s. One of the greatest obstacles was that we did not yet have the Internet, so the information that did exist and the experts who could help us were hard to find.

Today we have the opposite situation, with so much information that it is challenging to sort one's way through it all. And while there are some similarities, the reality is that each autistic child's situation is different from others. There are so many genes, environmental influences, and bodily processes that may be involved that how they manifest in one child is often quite different from how they show up in another.

The most important wisdom I have gained in this journey is to trust yourself and your knowledge of your child. Follow your heart and your intuition. No one knows your child as well as you do, and no one notices all the subtle reactions and signs as much as you. Be your child's loving and tenacious advocate.

Trust your child, too. They have reasons for their actions and reactions, which might be their attempts to communicate in nontraditional ways.

Resources
"What is Autism Spectrum Disorder?" CDC/Centers for Disease Control and Prevention
https://www.cdc.gov/ncbddd/autism/facts.html

"Signs and Symptoms of Autism Spectrum Disorders," CDC/ Centers for Disease Control and Prevention
https://www.cdc.gov/ncbddd/autism/signs.html

"Autism Spectrum Disorder Fact Sheet," National Institute of Neurological Disorders and Stroke/National Institutes of Health (NIH)
https://www.ninds.nih.gov/Disorders/Patient-Caregiver-Education/ Fact-Sheets/Autism-Spectrum-Disorder-Fact-Sheet

"What Is Autism Spectrum Disorder?"
American Psychiatric Association
https://www.psychiatry.org/patients-families/autism/ what-is-autism-spectrum-disorder

"Understanding Autism," Autism Society
https://autismsociety.org/the-autism-experience/

"Signs of Autism in Babies: A Simple Guide to Developmental Differences," Healthline - March 19, 2021
https://www.healthline.com/health/autism/ signs-of-autism-in-babies

"What Are Signs of Autism in Infants?" PsychCentral, December 21, 2021
https://psychcentral.com/autism/signs-of-autism-in-infants

THE WHITE BINDER

In the mid-1990s and earlier, it was very difficult for parents to find information, or even knowledgeable doctors or other parents, to help them when their child was diagnosed with autism. Some parents and experts had, in fact, studied the issue very deeply and written books about it, but they were not easy to learn about. The Internet was just developing and not available for the general public. Most people did not have personal computers, components such as modems were extremely slow and rudimentary, and there were no cellphones.

Dr. Bernard Rimland (1928-2006)
Dr. Bernard Rimland, spurred by the need to find ways to help his own autistic son, revolutionized the autism field by reconceptualizing it into a scientific biological approach and provided much-needed explanations and guidance to other parents searching for the same kinds of information. After publishing his groundbreaking book, *Infantile Autism: The Syndrome and Its Implications for a Neural Theory of Behavior*, he founded the Autism Society of America and the Autism Research Institute in San Diego.

Resource
Stephen M. Edelson, PhD., "In Memoriam: Bernard Rimland's 'Infantile Autism': The Book That Changed Autism," Autism Research Review International, Vo. 28, No. 1, 2014
https://www.autism.org/bernard-rimlands-infantile-autism/

Lifelines

The white binder was a lifeline to me in the mid-1990s when I began searching for information about autism and experts for guidance. Now in 2022 the vast number of resources available is both a blessing and yet often overwhelming, as well as challenging to evaluate. Listed below are some that will help you get started or deepen your understanding of what you already know.

Resources

The US Government provides a variety of information, resources, funding, programs and support through many agencies and departments, especially the Department of Health and Human Services. A coordinating page with an overview of federal programs regarding autism is: https://iacc.hhs.gov/resources/organizations/federal/

Highlights from this site include:

National Institute of Mental Health - Information on autism, including links to clinical trials, at https://www.nimh.nih.gov/health/topics/autism-spectrum-disorders-asd

Eunice Kennedy Shriver National Institute for Child Health and Human Development - https://www.nichd.nih.gov/health/topics/autism/clinicaltrials

Office of Early Childhood Development - A substantial collection of information, including evaluation and education services available under the Individuals with Disabilities Education Act (IDEA) - https://www.acf.hhs.gov/ecd/child-health-development/asd

Centers for Medicare and Medicaid Services - Options available for furnishing medical and therapy services - https://www.medicaid.gov/medicaid/benefits/autism-services/index.html

Many autism programs exist at universities and university hospitals that provide diagnostics, therapy, research, and clinical trials. Investigate what programs the universities in your area may have, or may be able to refer you to. There are likely to be many other autism clinics and service providers as well.

San Francisco Bay Area

Stanford Autism Center, Stanford Children's Health, Stanford - Provides specialized clinical services and advanced research in autism spectrum disorder, bringing together professionals across Stanford hospitals, departments and disciplines.
https://www.stanfordchildrens.org/en/service/autism

UC-Davis Health MIND Institute, Davis - The Institute's clinic provides assessments and treatment recommendations to providers as well as participation in clinical research studies, training for providers and researchers, resources and education.
https://health.ucdavis.edu/mindinstitute/

Southern California

Center for Autism Research & Treatment, UCLA, Los Angeles
https://www.semel.ucla.edu/autism

Koegel Autism Center, UC Santa Barbara, Santa Barbara - The center provides diagnostic assessments, intervention services, parent support, and clinical training opportunities, as well as providing research and clinical training to doctoral students in clinical psychology and special education.
https://education.ucsb.edu/autism

UC San Diego Autism Center of Excellence (ACE) - Developmental evaluations, research. https://neurosciences.ucsd.edu/centers-programs/autism/index.html

District of Columbia

Children's National Center for Autism Spectrum Disorders, Washington - Autism evaluation and treatment services, executive function and social skills groups, gender and autism program. https://childrensnational.org/departments/center-for-neuroscience-and-behavioral-medicine/programs-and-services/center-for-autism-spectrum-disorders

Florida

Johns Hopkins All Children's Hospital, Autism Program, St. Petersburg - Comprehensive assessment and diagnostic services, outpatient therapy sessions, caregiver education, behavioral parent training services, books, and educational material. https://www.hopkinsallchildrens.org/Services/Autism-Center

Iowa

University of Iowa Stead Family Children's Hospital, Iowa City - Team evaluation diagnosis, medication management, behavior assessment, early intervention, issue evaluations. https://uichildrens.org/medical-services/autism

Maryland

University of Maryland Children's Hospital, Baltimore - Diagnosis; therapies in behavioral management, cognitive behavior, education and school-based, joint attention, medication, nutritional, occupational, parent-mediated, physical, speech-language; social skills training; transitioning to adult.
https://www.umms.org/childrens/health-services/
behavioral-developmental-pediatrics/autism

Massachusetts and New England

Boston Children's Hospital, Autism Spectrum Center - Diagnostic evaluation, neurologic and development evaluations, management of ASD symptoms, specialty care, recommendations and referrals, assistance, speech and language evaluations and treatments, medication management and consultations, occupational and physical therapy, research studies.
https://www.childrenshospital.org/programs/
autism-spectrum-center-program

Massachusetts General Hospital, Alan and Lorraine Bressler Clinical and Research Program for Autism Spectrum Disorder, Boston - Comprehensive psychiatric assessments, care plans, medications, research studies.
https://www.massgeneral.org/psychiatry/treatments-and-services/
clinical-and-research-program-for-autism-spectrum-disorder

Missouri

Southeast Missouri State University, University Autism Center, Cape Girardeau
https://semo.edu/autism-center/

Washington University School of Medicine in St. Louis, Autism Clinical Center - Diagnosis and comprehensive intervention planning, applied behavior analysis and positive behavior support plans, psychiatric intervention.
https://childpsychiatry.wustl.edu/clinical-services/autismcenter/

New York

New York-Presbyterian Center for Autism and the Developing Brain - Affiliated with Weill Cornell Medicine and Columbia University - Diagnostic testing and evaluation, behavioral programming, occupational and speech therapy, medical services, social skills, family education, parent support groups.
https://www.nyp.org/psychiatry/
center-for-autism-the-developing-brain

Ohio

University Hospitals Rainbow Babies & Children's Hospital's Division of Developmental and Behavioral Pediatrics and Psychology, Cleveland - Autism diagnostic clinic, consultation with families, accessing behavioral therapies, integrating education and support services, transition to adulthood for teens.
https://www.uhhospitals.org/rainbow/services/
pediatric-developmental-and-behavioral-issues/autism

Utah

University of Utah Huntsman Mental Health Institute Autism Spectrum Disorder Clinic, Salt Lake City - Assessments, social skill and recreational groups, individual/family therapy, Parent Child Interaction Therapy (PCIT), behavior intervention, early intervention services, parent training, research.
https://healthcare.utah.edu/hmhi/treatments/autism-clinic/

Washington

Seattle Children's Hospital, Research, Foundation - Autism Center - Diagnostic evaluation, therapies for challenging behaviors, treatments and services, research, and clinical trials
https://www.seattlechildrens.org/clinics/autism-center/

Local and regional organizations often provide specialized information and resources for specific areas, such as the San Francisco Autism Society for the Bay Area.
https://sfautismsociety.org

THE BOY IN THE ROOM

Applied Behavior Analysis, behavioral therapists, and occupational therapists are covered in the glossary.

HOPE

Prompts and drills are covered in the glossary.

CHILDREN'S WORK

Dr. Pamela Wolfberg and Dr. Adriana Schuler -
Integrated Play Groups

Dr. Pamela Wolfberg and Dr. Adriana Schuler, both at San Francisco State University, collaborated on the development of the Integrated Play Groups model. Early in her career, Dr. Wolfberg recognized that children with autism did not play the kinds of social and imaginary games that their neurotypical classmates engaged in. Rather, they were more likely to engage in unique and narrowly focused activities that left them out of opportunities for learning social interactions and gaining confidence by being part of social groups.

So, she, joined by Dr. Schuler, developed the Integrated Play Groups, which brought together neurotypical and autistic children to co-create an inclusive play culture that fosters social engagement and creative expression. The groups were designed to take place in natural settings— school, home, outdoors—with the help of trained adult playgroup guides. The guides' responsibility was to encourage integrated play with all the children and to guide them, when necessary, to find ways to join their interests in order to return to collaborative shared activities.

All the children learned in these playgroup settings. The children with autism developed more socially coordinated and representational forms of play, while the neurotypical children gained empathy and relationship-building skills.

Resources
Pamela Wolfberg, et al., "Including Children with Autism in Social and Imaginary Play with Typical Peers: Integrated Play Groups Model," American Journal of Play, Fall 2012
https://files.eric.ed.gov/fulltext/EJ985604.pdf

Autism Collective for Peer Socialization, Play and Imagination
http://wolfberg.com

Anna Jean Ayres (1920-1988) - Ayres Sensory Integration

Dr. A. Jean Ayres was an occupational therapist, psychologist, and neuroscientist who developed a therapy approach for children with disabilities, including autism, that built upon developing stronger sensory awareness. Through strengthening sensory perceptions received through our bodies—including sight, sound, hearing, taste, touch, body position, balance, and movement— we form a more accurate assessment of our environment. This heightened sensory awareness, in turn, allows us to make realistic and adaptive plans and responses to self-care, social participation, and other situations. It also assists in creating an awareness of steps to accomplish tasks, along with more intricate motor actions.

Children on the autism spectrum often have difficulties or sensitivities to many sensory inputs, such as bright lights or loud noises. They might have an awkward sense of balance. The feel or sound of brushing their teeth might be problematic. These kinds of difficulties can make typical environments or groups —including classes or even families— seem overwhelming to them. Occupational therapists can help identify these challenges and find ways to teach and adapt skills to make them more successful for the child.

Resources
About Ayres Sensory Integration
https://www.cl-asi.org/about-ayres-sensory-integration

Frequently Asked Questions About Ayres Sensory Integration
https://www.aota.org/-/media/Corporate/Files/Practice/Children/Resources/FAQs/SI%20Fact%20Sheet%202.pdf

MIRRORING

Dr. Stanley Greenspan (1941-2010) - Floortime

Dr. Stanley Greenspan believed that it was essential to treat the whole child, not just discrete specific behaviors, and that emotions are the integrating factor for human development. Communication and emotional health, in fact, he said, are the keys to becoming more emotionally mature—for any child or adult, not just those with autism.

He developed Floortime in collaboration with Dr. Serena Wieder. Floortime is a relationship-based therapy that focuses on the child's interests and builds on their strengths. The therapist or parent follows the child's lead and enters their games, expanding on emotional back-and-forth exchanges, called Circles of Communication, that stimulate the development of the child's brain circuitry.

Resources
https://www.stanleygreenspan.com

SPECIAL CHILDREN

Why Is Autism Increasing?

In 2018, the US Centers for Disease Control and Prevention (CDC) reported that 1 in 44 8-year-old children had autism. Boys were 4.2 times more likely to be diagnosed with autism than girls. The CDC began tracking the prevalence of ASD in 1996. In 2000 and 2002, ASD estimates were 6.7 (one in 150) per one thousand 8-year-old children. In 2016, it had increased to 18.5 (one in 54).

Below are popular theories that try to explain the increase in autism:

1) Evolving criteria - In 1994, the American Psychiatric Association (APA) recognized autism for the first time in their Diagnostic and Statistical Manual of Mental Disorders (DSM-IV), expanding the levels of autism that might be diagnosed. In 2013, the APA released DSM-5, which folded Asperger and other diagnostic autism levels into one category, allowing more people to fit the definition.

2) Changes in reporting methods

3) Possible environmental factors, including later parental ages, air pollution or pesticides, maternal health, extreme prematurity or low birth rate, and incidences of oxygen deprivation during birth.

Scientific American presented more considerations in interpreting the CDC data:

4) The CDC relies on "snapshots" from eleven data sites around the country and may have previously missed children who did not have school or medical records.

5) Increasing awareness of autism - Until the 1980s, they report, many people with autism were institutionalized, making them essentially invisible.
6) Greater accuracy in diagnosis and reporting.

7) Advantages of getting an autism diagnosis to qualify for specialized services and special education, when in the past those were not available.

Resources
https://www.cdc.gov/mmwr/volumes/70/ss/ss7011a1.htm

https://www.verywellhealth.com/
is-there-a-real-increase-in-the-incidence-of-autism-260133

https://www.scientificamerican.com/article/
the-real-reasons-autism-rates-are-up-in-the-u-s/

PRIVILEGED

Who funds special education?

Much of the burden for educating children with autism falls on the
school systems as well as on parents. Some states have adopted laws
that mandate insurance providers fund some therapies. This varies
by state and provider.

The education code is complex, which is the reason why some
parents choose to seek the help of an advocate or an education
attorney. Although these avenues may be expensive, there are legal
advocates that provide pro-bono services. Check with the Legal
Aid Society in your area to find pro-bono services. Below are laws
that outline the rights of individuals with disabilities:

IDEA - Individuals with Disabilities Education Act is the law
that makes available a free appropriate public education to
eligible children with disabilities throughout the nation.

FAPE - Free and Appropriate Public Education is the cornerstone
of IDEA defining the specifics of the terms outlined in the law,
appropriate education and modifications, aids, and related services
free of charge to students with disabilities and their parents or
guardians. The "appropriate" component means that this education
must be designed to meet the individual educational needs of the
student as determined through appropriate evaluation and placement procedures.

Each state provides services for individuals with disabilities. Parent support networks are helpful in providing contact information for state resources.

Resources
About IDEA
https://sites.ed.gov/idea/#

Sec. 300.101 Free appropriate public education (FAPE)
https://sites.ed.gov/idea/regs/b/b/300.101

OUT OF SYNC

One way to cope with emotional pain.

I came to know myself in a deeper way by understanding my personality. In the process I learned how my coping strategies had helped me confront the truth about my son's diagnosis. The Enneagram became a guide to understanding my coping strategies and protective mechanisms.

Resource
Howe-Murphy, Roxanne. Deep Living with the Enneagram: Recovering Your True Nature (Revised and Updated). Enneagram Press. Kindle Edition.

KNOWING THE UNKNOWN

The Enneagram became a map that helped me understand the underlying patterns that had unconsciously guided me through my life.

Resource

"The primary reason for working with the Enneagram is to help us awaken to our true nature. It puts us on a path of healing and real transformation that, for most of us, takes place over time—with patience, trust, faith in our awakening journey—and by being as present as possible."

Howe-Murphy, Roxanne. Deep Living with the Enneagram: Recovering Your True Nature (Revised and Updated). Enneagram Press. Kindle Edition.

THREE MARRIAGES

Wings Learning Center evolved into a Non-Public School certified by the California Department of Education. It continues to serve children who are severely impacted by autism. In 2022, the school serves children and adults around the San Francisco Bay Area on its campus in Redwood City, California.

ATONAL SYMPHONY

Talker, Lightwriter, and AAC Devices

Augmentative communication (AAC) devices are often introduced to non-verbal individuals by a speech therapist in a home or school setting. As technology has evolved, augmentative communication devices such as tablets, laptops, and smartphones have become more widely used. Aaron continues to use an outdated AAC device called the Lightwriter. We referred to it as his Talker.

Circles of Communication

Opening and closing circles of communication is a way of naturally interacting with one another. A person reaches out with a look, gesture, sound, or word, and then another person responds, building on the initial action. This is referred to as opening and closing a circle of communication. The Relational Development Intervention (RDI) and Floortime Models use this communicative intent as a cornerstone of their therapeutic approach.

Resource
The Interdisciplinary Council on Development and Learning
https://www.icdl.com

POLARITIES

9/11

On September 11, 2001, nineteen attackers associated with al-Qaeda, an Islamic extremist group, hijacked four airplanes from commercial airports. Two were flown into the World Trade Center in New York City, which soon collapsed, killing 2,750 people. Another plane flew into the Pentagon outside Washington, DC, killing 184 people. A fourth plane crashed in rural Pennsylvania, killing forty people, after the passengers fought for control of the plane. All the hijackers died in the crashes. In New York, many of the dead were police and firefighters who had rushed into the World Trade Center and died when they fell. The U. S. population was in shock at the fact that the country had been successfully attacked, something that seemed impossible on such an audacious and large scale before 9/11.

Resource
https://www.britannica.com/event/September-11-attacks/
The-September-11-commission-and-its-findings

A VIEW FROM THE KITCHEN TABLE

Parents need a community of support around them, and this is especially important when there are so many new and often unexpected things to learn and challenging decisions to make. That is true in almost all parenting situations, but particularly when raising a child with autism.

It is important, both for your child and also for yourself, not to become isolated. You need support and love both for yourself, and also to best help your child. The group I found most helpful in the Bay Area was Parents Helping Parents in San Jose, CA (https://www.php.com).

There are many local parents' groups all around the country. Your doctor, the clinic that may have evaluated your child, or an autism clinic at a local university or hospital are good places to start for suggestions.

DEAR DR. SCHULER

Adriana Schuler had a profound effect on my life as well as on Aaron's. She collaborated on developing Integrated Play Groups, teaching that play is how children develop the skills they need for their futures. She planted the seeds for Wings and guided the educators on how to implement a new approach for children with autism. She sent the perfect person to be Aaron's aide and teacher in a new school. And then she left way too soon.

PECS

The Picture Exchange Communication System (PECS) teaching protocol is based on B.F. Skinner's book, Verbal Behavior, and broad spectrum (ABA) applied behavior analysis.

PECS consists of six phases and begins by teaching an individual to give a single picture of a desired item or action to a "communicative partner" who immediately honors the exchange as a request. The system goes on to teach discrimination of pictures and how to put them together in sentences. In the more advanced phases, individuals are taught to use modifiers, answer questions, and comment.

Resources
Dr. Barry Prizant and Dr. Pamela Wolfberg, both close collaborators with Dr. Adriana Schuler, wrote this beautiful memorial to her.
https://www.sfsu.edu/~autism/In%20Memory%20of%20
Adriana%20Loes%20Schuler.pdf

What is PECS?
https://pecs.com/picture-exchange-communication-system-pecs/

UNRESTRAINED EXCHANGE

Epilepsy and Autism

Epilepsy is known to occur in a higher-than-expected proportion of individuals with autism. Epilepsy is often referred to as a comorbidity.

It may be that individuals with epilepsy are at higher risk for aggressive behavior only when they also have impaired executive functions.

Programs for first responders

As Aaron became more at ease among larger groups of people it became important for his caregivers to be aware of how to handle behaviors that may appear violent. Across the country programs have been created to provide training not only to people with disabilities and their caregivers, but also to first responders, and other members of the community.

Resources
Epilepsy and Autism: Is There a Relationship?
https://www.epilepsy.com/article/2017/3/
epilepsy-and-autism-there-relationship

National Institute of Neurological Disorders and Stroke (NINDS)
https://magazine.medlineplus.gov/article/
understanding-different-kinds-of-seizures/

Center for Decease Control and Prevention - National resources for first responders
https://www.cdc.gov/ncbddd/disabilityandhealth/emergency-tools.
html#forfirstresponders

TEA TIME

Zoloft and Abilify

Zoloft (generic: sertraline) and Abilify (generic: aripiprazole) are each often prescribed for autism anxiety symptoms. They work differently from each other and have different benefits and side effects.

Resources:
Overviews
https://www.drugs.com/compare/abilify-vs-zoloft
https://psychcentral.com/autism/medications-for-autism#ssr-is

ONE BREATH AT A TIME

What does the body have to do with it?

My body as a source of information was foreign to me, until
I began to experience the impact of "getting into my body" through
yoga, breathing, and somatic practices. Knowing and sensing
into the sensations that were present when I was feeling stressed
supported me through some very difficult times. By learning to
connect with the sensations in my body, I was able to distinguish
between real and perceived threats, to me and my son.

Resources
"A direct experience is radically different. It is not filtered through
our mental processing or emotional upsets, but instead is sensed in
the body. Having a direct experience takes our attention below the
level of ideas and below the circumstances surrounding a situation.
We shift our focus from the obvious entanglements of the situation
and focus on what we might consider very unusual territory—what
is happening within our bodies. Here, in the sensations conveyed
through the body, we discover a whole new source of information
about ourselves, and about what contributes to our personality's
usual strategies."

Howe-Murphy, Roxanne. Deep Living with the Enneagram: Recovering Your True Nature (Revised and Updated). Enneagram Press. Kindle Edition.

"Our brain captures the strategies that work to keep us as safe, connected, and respected as possible in our early life environment, and then puts those behaviors on autopilot. Just like getting the spoon to your mouth."

Blake, Amanda. Your Body is Your Brain: Leverage Your Somatic Intelligence to Find Purpose, Build Resilience, Deepen Relationships and Lead More Powerfully (p. 19). Embright, LLC. Kindle Edition.

THE STEP YOU DON'T WANT TO TAKE

Belinda Gore's life changed in 1984 when she began working with anthropologist Felicitas Goodman who taught her the art of ritual postures.

Dr. Felicitas Goodman, a cultural anthropologist and linguist who spoke and wrote eight languages, joined a groundbreaking study when her mentor, cultural anthropologist Erika Bourguignon, hired her to translate hundreds of ethnographies collected in a National Institute of Mental Health survey of indigenous cultures worldwide.

Resources
The Cuyamungue Institute
https://www.cuyamungueinstitute.com

WHEN I'M GONE

Living Communities

Between 2014 and 2016, I visited four living communities and met with the individuals whose passion and commitment to the well-being of the residents are clearly seen on the faces of those they serve.

Misericordia, Chicago, IL https://www.misericordia.com
Libenu, Chicago IL https://www.libenu.org
FCSN, Fremont, CA https://fcsn1996.org
Clearwater Ranch, Cloverdale, CA https://www.cranch.net

About the Author

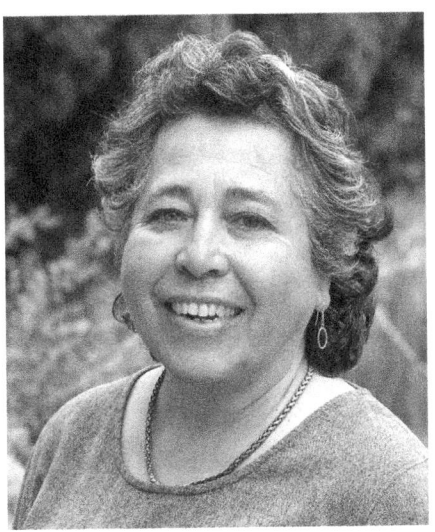

Irma Velasquez was born and raised in El Salvador and immigrated to the San Francisco Bay area in the early 60s. Her son's unexpected diagnosis of autism moved her to address a gap in the education system and social services for underserved youth. She launched a school for children with autism and designed creative programs for young adults of different abilities. Her memoir is inspired by her love for her son, her dedication to her community, and her passion for art.

Irma is a social entrepreneur and an artist and advocate, inspiring social change through the power of self-expression, social engagement, and inner awareness.

Made in the USA
Monee, IL
11 October 2022

15657964R00148